Pathways to Success: Training for Independent Living

**Monographs of the American
Association
on Mental Retardation, 15**

Michael J. Begab, Series Editor

Pathways to Success: Training for Independent Living

by

Steven H. Stumpf
University of Southern California

Published by
American Association on Mental Retardation
1719 Kalorama Road, NW
Washington, DC 20009

No. 15, Monographs of the American Association on Mental Retardation (ISSN 0895-8009)

Library of Congress Cataloging-in-Publication Data

Stumpf, Steven H., 1949–
   Pathways to success: training for independent living / by Steven H. Stumpf.
   p. cm. — (Monographs of the American Association on Mental Retardation: 15)
   Includes bibliographical references.
   ISBN 0-940898-25-X: $22.95
   1. Mentally handicapped—Housing—United States—Case studies. 2. Mentally handicapped—Rehabilitation—United States—Case studies. I. Title. II. Series.
HV3006.A4S79 1990
363.5'974—dc20   90-23888
                                                                 CIP

Printed in the United States of America

Table of Contents

Foreword

I don't know whether I am unusual or not, but I know that my own qualitative research with mentally retarded adults, in which I delve into many of the intimate and closely held aspects of their everyday lives, leaves me slightly shaken. There are two reasons for this. The first is that, no matter how many times I have done this in the past, I am always unexpectedly humbled at being granted the opportunity to record the little and grand successes and failures that happen to people, whether labeled retarded or not, with whom I am doing participant-observation research, but who, in the final analysis, I do not know all that well. The sense of trust and openness that flows in successful fieldwork from "study participant" to "researcher" (and, in the very best experience of fieldwork, in the opposite direction as well) gives me the sense, certainly, of gratification, but of responsibility as well.

My second reason for being shaken during fieldwork seems particularly related to doing research with mildly retarded adults. To a very large extent, researchers and service providers approach their various tasks with retarded adults with one major and usually, I think, unexamined assumption: these people, and the lives they create for themselves, are not normal. In fact, the law requires that we *provide* retarded adults *normalizing experiences* in *least restrictive environments*. If *we* have to *do* this *for* them, there must be something wrong with them, since they can't get it (whatever *it* is) for themselves. Elsewhere we have noted the association in our collective unconscious between mildly retarded individuals and other infantilized populations: criminals, women, people with mental illnesses, and stone age savages (Langness & Levine, 1986). Such people are also not (or, in the case of Western children, not *quite*) normal. Of course, when asked, many of us who <u>are</u> *normal* would agree that, upon reflection, it seems impossible to define normalcy. What astounds me is that, when dealing with the mildly retarded individuals of our society, we can and do make many decisions, not so much about what is normal, but about what is normal *enough*. What would it take for the little messes and contradictions in my life to be considered not normal *enough* ?

I do not raise this issue about normalcy and its definition because I am about to engage in an extended diatribe on the indignities and injustices of *the system*. Others have already made thoughtful and convincing arguments along these lines. Rather, I raise the issue because I do think that, before proceeding much farther in our research or reflection, we are obliged to challenge our sloppy thinking about concepts such as normalcy. And, as I see it, one of the best ways to disabuse ourselves of the static and unidimensional notions of normalcy and normal-enough that burden our scientific thinking is to surround ourselves with, among other things, sympathetic studies of the real, day-to-day lives of retarded persons. In these studies, moreover, their voices, as well as those of the others (parents, families, friends, case workers, etc.) who help create their lives, must be prominently featured. So, too, must the minutiae of daily life. The complete file of such minutiae—a necessary fiction, of course—may help us better appreciate the shifting and delicate nature of competence (and incompetence) in the world, our own commonalities with these struggles, the unrelenting pressures of being judged as competent or not (i.e., just *normal enough*), and the real injustice of having the struggles of one's life scrutinized, categorized, and, inevitably, trivialized.

Steven Stumpf's book, which you have before you, is a further, and significant, addition to this enterprise of building up our understanding of the daily lives of mildly mentally retarded individuals. His long-term research with his mildly retarded study participants, and his obvious rapport with the majority of them, has allowed him that deep look into the sometimes sad, sometimes comical, sometimes strategic, sometimes dumb, sometimes hearty, and sometimes subdued accommodations that they, like the rest of us, must make to life and one's own inner needs.

Stumpf's book does much more than this, however. It forces us to take the predictability out of our assumptions about retarded lives-in-process. Stumpf has shown us, as have other skilled qualitative researchers, that the "condition" or "state" or "success" of one's life depends upon who is doing the viewing. In this case, we hear the voices of family, friends, clinical staff, the retarded person him/herself, and Stumpf's own voice as both sympathetic observer, hard-nosed researcher, and clinician. Stumpf also prods us to think of success or failure not as a static or fixed outcome but rather as "a changing, variant, idiosyncratic event, a function of the individual in context of personal history and the learning environment". Through his accounts of these lives we can feel their ups and downs, occasioned by the complex, and unpredictable, rule of history, fortune, and innate ability. These lives—at least Stumpf's portrayal of them—are a grand disclaimer to the existence and power of individually-based or program-based predictor variables that are rendered, as other critics have noted, inexact and shifting.

Steven Stumpf's book also is a rare insider's account and evaluation of a small-scale independent living skills training program. The account of this "mom and pop" social service agency leaves one a little breathless and edgy. The program, with all its good intentions and early successes, suffers from staff burnout and turnover, questionable in-service training for staff, some administrative short-sightedness or lack of focus, and half-hearted evaluation practices. In a world where the primary objective is training others to be reasoning, thoughtful, planful human beings—in short, normal (we like to think)—

the emperor has no clothes. At least, so it seems. Perhaps the real message is that programs of this type have their successes and failures, too, and that whether you attribute one or the other to it depends upon your point of view and the time you observe. Certainly New Start's clients, the retarded adults being taught to be *normal*, found reason to both castigate and praise it.

This business of teaching people to act normally is itself a curiosity. Stumpf records for us the need for basic lessons in the basics: using the bus, cooking and cleaning, doing the laundry, shopping alone, constructing grocery lists or weekly calendars, social deportment, money management, and so forth. And program staff, I am sure, tried their damnedest to teach the right way to balance a checkbook, to shop economically, to plan the week. But that is just the problem: no one who already lives independently is very likely to do all of these things in all the *right* ways. What is missing from this, and the many other training programs that dot the landscape, is the cacophony of errors, fumblings, half-baked or half-hearted efforts, and indiscretions that describe life as lived. In their well-intentioned zealousness to act normally, both project staff and clients unwittingly subscribe to a standard of behavior that is decidedly abnormal. Most of us really live, as it were, between the cracks.

Insofar as training has an effect on clients—and Stumpf maintains that there is little relationship between skill teaching and learning, on the one hand, and success at independent living, on the other—it is to keep them away from the cracks and as afraid of falling into them as possible. Anxiety, fear of being exposed for what you *really* are, and an inability to play with and disregard, when necessary, the rules of everyday life would seem to be the most visible outcomes of independent living training programs such as is documented here.

Steven Stumpf's book is refreshingly readable, to the point, chock full of interesting personalities and psychopathologies, and thoughtful. For my money, however, its value is the accumulation of ethnographic accounts of real people and real lives struggling with the ongoing dilemmas of trying to be normal (not just *normal enough*) and successful in their everyday lives. It is the variety and interpretation of the human experience that is so endlessly fascinating and moving.

Harold G. Levine, Ph.D.
Associate Professor
Graduate School of Education
University of California, Los Angeles

Reference
Langness, L.L., and Levine, H.G. (1986). Introduction. *In culture and retardation: Life histories of mildly retarded persons in American society* (L.L. Langness & H.G. Levine, Eds.), pp.ix-xv. Dordrecht: D. Reidel Publishing Company.

Introduction

Over the previous 30 years, the field of mental retardation has produced much real-world drama: shifts in philosophy; upheavals in state and local systems of care; heated debate on appropriate methods for treatment and service; and, inevitably, an increase in knowledge and understanding.

These tumultuous developments were long coming. Although from their very inception the institutions that housed many retarded persons (known as public residential facilities, or PRFs) were intended to train, educate, and rehabilitate people with retardation for their return to the community, these intentions were compromised by a strong social sentiment to isolate this segment of the population.

The current trend toward community integration of persons with mental retardation is generally considered to coincide with the deinstitutionalization thrust of the Nixon Administration in the late 1960s. As PRFs became populated by individuals with more severe forms of handicap, some states began to extend community placements to the less severely retarded (especially the mildly retarded) in foster and family work settings. Only in the past 10 to 15 years has placement been extended on any significant scale to the severely and profoundly retarded as well. For the most part, these groups have been relocated in small group homes, foster family homes, Intermediate Care Facilities (ICFs), or nursing homes.

The 15 individuals reported on in this study have a borderline or mild disability or are emotionally disturbed. Their personality profiles seem quite different from their mildly retarded counterparts admitted to institutions 30 to 40 years ago. It would seem, therefore, that their lives following graduation from independent living training would have little to do with issues related to deinstitutionalization. Yet the fact that none of them have experienced institutional life is a consequence of the deinstitutionalization movement, as is most certainly the philosophy that underlies the independent living training movement.

The vast majority of people with mental retardation, as far as professionals in the field and interested lay persons are concerned, are a "hidden" population. Throughout history, well under 10 percent (depending on the definition) of the mentally retarded have ever known institutions. With IQ tests in increasing disfavor and more children being mainstreamed, identification of this population will become even more difficult. We should recognize that persons with mental retardation are by definition impaired in their adaptive behavior. In fact, a major cause for placement of people with mild retardation in institutions after failure to adjust in the community has been maladaptive behavior.

Many early studies on community adaptation of people with mild retardation were conducted with subjects who had been previously institutionalized for varying periods of time. These subjects constituted for the most part a select group, as they came from the lowest social class and often exhibited behavior that was either antisocial, unlawful, or otherwise unacceptable to the community. Their subsequent return to the institution was generally not attributable to low intelligence. The institutional regimen may not have readily prepared them for independent decision making in a less structured environment.

It is a paradox of our field that most of our knowledge is derived from studies of institutional groups. In the behavioral sciences the wards have provided excellent laboratories for testing and developing behavior modification techniques and programs. Even biomedical research, at least those studies involving human subjects closely monitored by Human Experimentation Committees, has benefited greatly from the captive population and controlled environment these facilities provide.

Undoubtedly, much of what we have learned regarding factors influencing adaptive placement of people with mild retardation in the community could be generalized to those who were never institutionalized. Still, selective elements, such as the need for medical supervision and behavior management, can provide meaningful discriminating variables, as can differences in family resources and coping skills and also the experience of institutionalization.

How might these variables bear on the independent living training curriculum for these conceivably different groups? How can preexistent training in skills from the institution or family affect the curriculum? In evaluating the effectiveness of a community training program, should expectations be the same regardless of individual backgrounds?

It is beyond the scope of this monograph to address all of these questions. They are raised in part to draw attention to the limited knowledge available on that very large segment of the retarded population living in marginal and unobserved circumstances. The reader is cautioned to consider these points when interpreting the pathways trod by the subjects in this study—the paved roads and potholes they have encountered on the route to success or failure.

As a result of the deinstitutionalization/normalization/community placement movement, many programs for people with mild mental retardation are now available from the earliest years. More and more mildly retarded individuals are systematically enrolled in education, training, and rehabilitation programs that culminate in independent living following many years of effort.

Many of these placement efforts have narrowly judged success in terms of the graduates' ability not to return to their families' homes.

Correspondingly, evaluation has narrowly assessed training effects, typically in terms of the return rate. These criteria are simply too limited and have yielded little understanding as to whether and how the mildly retarded might best be assisted to live in the community.

This study, then, is an attempt to understand on a no-larger-than-life-size-scale how independent living training has been realized in the lives of 15 adults with mild retardation. Their involvement in and subsequent graduation from a training program, at one time considered to be the apex for such programs, is examined from the perspectives of several "stakeholders" in the participants' successful training. Much is learned about the nature of such programs (which are often created and implemented at the local level) and about criteria more useful and illuminating for determining success and failure than the return rate alone.

In the course of this study two contributions have been made concerning research on people with mild mental retardation. First, in order for the body of information on this population to be substantially and meaningfully extended, a specific type of methodology must be employed; that is, the method of description employed herein, generically referred to as *qualitative* research. Second, one of the most widely advocated and employed strategies for preventing reinstitutionalization of this population has been independent living training. There has been much training but little program evaluation. Information is sparse on the practice and efficacy of independent living as it actually occurs in a community-based program for people with mild mental retardation. This study adds to the nascent body of work on independent living programs by demonstrating the utility of qualitative methods in understanding how the lives of those persons being trained to live on their own for the first time in the community are affected.

Chapter 1

The Qualitative Evaluation of Success

This study addresses three principle areas: a.) appropriate methodology for the evaluation of a growing class of community residential facilities called *Independent Living Skills Training Programs;* b.) the definition of success and failure for graduates of these programs; and c.) key factors that may contribute to the success of these programs as well as their graduates.

Based on results of this study, it will be argued that qualitative methods are best suited to the evaluation of small, "mom and pop" social service agencies that are operated on a shoestring budget with one or two key administrators and an all-too-often underqualified staff; that success and failure must be defined through the eyes of the participants along with the agency staff and family/friends that support them; and that psychosocial/ developmental factors such as the ability to make friends, and keep parents at a distance where they remain supportive yet separate, may be critical to an individual's success.

Community Residential Facilities (CRFs) and Public Residential Facilities (PRFs) refer to the two classes of residential facilities available to people with mental retardation in this country. CRFs are typically composed of board and care homes, foster family homes, older adult group homes, and apartment-placement programs. PRFs are the more traditional public institutions that, prior to the emergence of CRFs, were the primary form of care available to people with mental retardation. CRFs differ significantly from PRFs, not only in size, location, and other physical characteristics, but also in their philosophical approach to the treatment and care of people with mental retardation. The proliferation of CRFs as the facility of choice for people with mental retardation is based upon the belief that they can adapt and adjust to a normal community life, and should be presented with every opportunity to do so. The establishment of PRFs, by contrast, was motivated by sympathy, considered radical at the time, to both serve and protect that population, but well outside and preferably away from the "normal" community.

The current abundance of CRFs reflects a wide and major shift in public policy pertaining to the care and treatment of all special, marginal populations (e.g., people with mental illnesses, parolees, and people with mental retardation). This shift is rooted in the social turmoil of the 1960s, a time when many long-standing social policies were challenged. Until the '60s era, prevailing opinion held that these special populations were best kept apart from the broader society, where they could be humanely cared for in institutional settings. Critics claimed that the institutions were not humane, that they were disconnected from the mainstream of society and thereby obstructed habilitation. Habilitation, they argued, could take place more effectively in the community where opportunities for adjusting and adapting to community norms played key roles.

The sudden appearance of these facilities in large numbers and multiple forms coincided with the widespread acceptance of certain beliefs about people with mental retardation that at first glance seemed to depart radically from established beliefs. These new beliefs stated that: a.) people with mental retardation deserved opportunities equal to those enjoyed by the normal population; b.) they could benefit developmentally from these opportunities, subsequently enjoying a normal community life; and c.) society had a responsibility to provide the settings in which these opportunities could be encountered. CRFs were viewed as the manifest expression of these beliefs and as being fundamentally different from PRFs. It is ironic that PRFs were originally developed as alternative care facilities reflecting very similar beliefs.

The relative effectiveness of CRFs versus PRFs could not be determined via discussion involving the issues of philosophy and altruism alone. As was so common in the socially turbulent era of the 1960s, many programs were implemented based on the perceived correctness of their underlying social value.

Evaluation as an investigative tool emerged in response to the outcry from public and private arenas, which lobbied for the demonstrated effectiveness of these well-motivated programs.

Evaluation was the activity by which policy makers (i.e., legislators) sought to hold programs accountable for their intended goals. The initial conception of evaluation was closer to bookkeeping than to science. Evaluation as a field has since developed considerably, offering numerous approaches and encompassing a wide array of techniques in making assessments about program outcomes and operations.

Effectiveness is not limited to a dollar-and-cents analysis. Evaluation recognizes that the assessment of effectiveness varies with regard to the program's stage of development. The methods of analysis, therefore, may also vary accordingly.

The field of evaluation recently has been caught up in a struggle of rivalry in methodology. This methodological struggle has focused on the selection of techniques, quantitative or qualitative, to be employed when conducting program evaluation. Quantitative techniques are those of statistical analysis most commonly associated with experimental research and "hard science." Qualitative techniques are those of the descriptive analysis typically associated with "soft science." Concurrently, there has been similar controversy within research on CRFs and PRFs. It is not clear, after many years of research on habilitation of people with mental retardation, which variables or sets of variables should be selected for scrutiny in the evaluation of program effectiveness.

Recently, the controversies have overlapped in that the failure of research to demonstrate which variables are critical to program effectiveness has been linked to the predominant use of quantitative techniques, that is, experimentally based approaches. If qualitative methods were applied to the evaluation of CRFs, would a different set of factors, as well as a more illuminating body of information about the effectiveness of CRFs emerge?

This investigation utilized predominantly qualitative methods in conducting an evaluation of a vanguard CRF apartment-placement program for people with mental retardation, Project New Start, which trained them to live independently. Rather than conducting an in-depth investigation of program operations to help assess the program outcomes, this evaluation used the perspective of the graduates and a select group of peripherally involved people (e.g., program staff, graduates' family members, etc.), as well as documented program data that were available to the investigator, to describe the program and the ways in which the graduates did or did not achieve independent living. The rich descriptions of independent living from the viewpoints of related cohorts provides a framework for defining success—of the individuals and, by inference, of the program. Several factors that are underreported in this literature (e.g., friendship, familial interrelationships, the presence of family dysfunction and psychopathology) are brought out as significant contributors to the likelihood of success, and, therefore, as programmatic issues in so-called independent living skills training programs.

Success, as expressed in a quantified formula, is a fixed and dependent outcome of well-defined variables whose variances can be expressed as a mathematical relationship. For example, social science research has demonstrated the predictability of success (measured by income or career type) as a function of numerous factors, including spouse's income, parents' education, parents' employment, and so forth.

In the real lives of these sample members, however, success is a temporary condition that is varied and independent. It is not easily defined nor is it an apparent function of anything that has widespread predictability in the normal population. In fact, the entire world of the developmentally delayed does not seem to correspond readily to the world studied by most social science researchers. As the descriptions of these individuals' lives will bear out, success is a highly variable phenomenon, influenced by factors that are not easily understood.

There is a constant tendency by the observer to impose values from normal living in an effort to understand or predict behavior of the sample members. For the most part, these anticipatory predictions and expectations are misleading. By first following a rigorous observation style of recording as much as possible and then trying to explain what was witnessed after much data have been gathered, the different kinds of success, the varying levels within each kind, and the personal and family psychological dynamics that may contribute to success are revealed.

This approach also provided an unobtrusive measure of program effectiveness. It seemed that this approach would be better-suited to the evaluation of small social service programs, which have inaccurate records, high rates of staff turnover, poor documentation of program goals and objectives, and virtually no internal evaluation mechanisms.

Quantitative research predominates in the areas of program evaluation and independent living for people with mental retardation. As with all quantitative work, investigators of independent living and community adjustment have attempted to generate probability models that forecast adaptation outcomes based upon the skillful isolation of personal and/or programmatic variables demonstrated to have predictive value.

In the review of these investigations that follows, the failure of quantitative investigations to discover meaningful predictor variables is thoroughly summarized. This lack of success has in turn led some investigators (e.g., Bercovici, 1981, 1983; Edgerton, 1967, 1988; Sullivan et al., 1988) to argue that this model for research is ineffective, especially when compared with ethnographic methodologies, in promoting an understanding of those phenomena that describe the community adaptation and independent living of retarded adults. These same authors have stated that understanding is preceded by description and that description must begin as Bogdan and Taylor (1976) have advised, with "beliefs suspended."

Participant observation provides a rigorous method for systematically investigating the phenomenon of successful independent living. Participant observation is a method for gaining an insider's view of a given phenomenon. It requires that the researcher enter into the experience of the participant as openly as possible.

Once immersed in the participant's daily activities, the observer becomes like a participant himself while remaining an observer, carefully and unobtrusively making a record of the participant's actions. The method can be supplemented by interviews with the participant to document the intentions and motivations of the participant's behavior. The participant observer successively narrows the scope of the observations, moving from general to specific activities in the participant's life.

The participant observer seeks a richly detailed cultural description of the everyday life of a given group—in this case, those persons deemed successful graduates of Project New Start. The New Start staff as well as other peripherally related groups such as family members and adjunct service agency staff comprised a secondary source of informants.

Moreover, the program structure was also considered a source, in that it was specifically designed with certain features intended to facilitate independent living. The methods of participant observation (i.e., structured field observations documented by coded notes, and informal interviews) were used with the intent of providing a cross-section of views on the successful lives of the subjects.

Success is regularly assumed to be central to the evaluation of a program's worth, but in the case of the successful community adaptation of people with mental retardation, the concept of success itself is neither understood nor easily measured. The role of friendships and family involvement cannot be ignored in the program plan. The use of participant observation techniques offers a promising alternative in understanding this complex social phenomenon.

A Retrospective History of the Development, Investigation, and Evaluation of CRFs

Chapter 2

The Development of CRFs

It is useful to recount briefly how the treatment and care of marginal sectors of the population developed in this nation. Prior to the mid-1800s criminals were placed in penal colonies, while the insane and "feebleminded" were left to society's whims. Rejoining the community was not a goal. This view eventually succumbed to the belief that a responsible society would provide its less fortunate citizens with more humane treatment as well as hope for a better life. Humane treatment meant providing for the health care of these people while offering them rehabilitation programs. PRFs emerged as the locations where such would take place.

Viewed as idyllic settings of care and habilitation, PRFs aspired to provide "misfits" with a chance to become "normal." Unfortunately, these sites became institutions—final destinations rather than stopovers. They resembled little towns, practically self-sufficient, supporting two populations: the transient staff and the permanent residents. The hope they intended to offer to their residents (as departure points into the community) bred controversy within the community and quickly subverted their humanitarian intents:

> Their original intent to habilitate the mentally retarded was often frustrated by parent, professional and public pressures to prevent reentry of the handicapped into the community. . .the physical plant was designed for custodial care (Heal, Sigelman, & Switzky, 1978).

Resistance to placement of people with mental retardation in the community has been a recurring problem. The strongest prejudices have held that, once admitted to the community free of supervision, they would quickly fall into maladaptive behavior patterns. Vagrancy, unwanted pregnancy, destitution, and violence were predicted. These fears helped to keep the retarded in the institutions.

As a result, the PRF population grew steadily until 1967, when there were approximately 200,000 persons with mental retardation residing in public institutions. At this point a steady decline began. By 1978 there were 150,000 PRF residents, a 25 percent reduction.

This decrease can be directly attributed to the major social policy shift of the 1960s, in which issues of independence and accountability touched all segments of the population and affected all styles of life. New beliefs about this particular population's rights and abilities followed, indirectly encouraging the establishment of CRFs. These beliefs helped to overcome what Lakin, Bruininks, and Sigford (1981) referred to as the "cycle of persistent concerns" about people with mental retardation.

Despite evidence to the contrary, concerns about the dangers of allowing people with retardation to live unsupervised in the community have been persistently held by the general population. The first evidence that public fears might be exaggerated arose from a benchmark study by Fernald (1919), who reported on the community success of 568 residents released from the Massachusetts School for the Feebleminded between 1890 and 1914. Fernald was known as "one of the strongest supporters of segregation and...the social menace conception of the mentally retarded" (Heal et al., 1978). By defining success as being "at liberty" and "giving no trouble," Fernald reported a 53.6 percent success rate.

Deeply affected by his findings, Fernald joined that era's few advocates of community placement for the retarded. However, despite his own conclusion that the retarded could be safely released into the community, a finding that was concurrently supported by the reports of others (Anderson, 1922; Fernald, 1924; Wallace, 1929; Wallin, 1924), institutionalization held fast. An opposition movement, however, had begun.

Signs that the community placement movement was gaining momentum can be seen in the related social experiments that followed in the next two decades. Foster care homes, institutional parole plans for people with mental retardation, and a colony system (segregated farming facilities in the countryside) for selected residents were available to a limited degree in the '30s and '40s. After the Second World War a national parents' group emerged (the National Association for Retarded Children) as a strong advocacy union supporting dignified and humane treatment, especially in the form of institutional release.

However, the pivotal development of the community placement movement occurred in the '70s with the formulation of two ideological positions (*normalization* and the *developmental model*) and one legal doctrine (*least restrictive environment*). Together these concepts triggered the large-scale institutional release of adults with mental retardation into the community and ensured wider public acceptance.

The doctrine of normalization (Nirje, 1976; Wolfensberger, 1972) stated that people with mental retardation should have made available to them the patterns and conditions of everyday life that are typically available to the "normal" population. The developmental model of human growth as applied to people with mental retardation asserted that, given a normalization policy, people with mental retardation would be able to "develop," eventually exceeding present functional levels and as a result adapting to society.

The legal precedent of least restrictive environment was considered to be equally important by Bruininks, Kudla, Hauber, Bradley, and Wieck (1981). This doctrine held that, in order for normalization to occur, an environment must be created that was itself normal, as nonsegregated and nonrestrictive as possible. CRFs provided the settings where these principles could be practiced.

Once it became clear that CRFs were the residential rule rather than the exception, the issue of community placement was supplanted by a new policy focus: the habilitation of people with mental retardation to a normal lifestyle. There were many opinions on how they might best be assisted in adapting to the community. For every opinion there seemed to be a program, and for every program there was a CRF to implement it. In the rush to serve, the development of CRFs has taken place haphazardly and without any discernible plan. One approach to tracing this unguided growth is to develop a typology of the various kinds of CRFs available to people with mental retardation.

Types of CRFs

CRFs appeared suddenly and rapidly. There is no obvious order or system that easily describes and organizes the vast array of CRFs available to people with mental retardation. The absence of a suitable or generally agreed upon taxonomy of CRFs is testimony to the maverick, spurting growth of the community adaptation movement. Growth easily outstripped the ability of any regulatory agency to bring order to the field. New facilities operated with a free hand in reference to program design and the implementation of normalization. It is therefore no surprise that wide variation exists within the universe of CRFs and their particular interpretations of *normalization* and *least restrictive environment*.

Little agreement can be found on what constitutes the best, or even a minimal, normalization program. There is no general model for the evaluation of normalization programs and their relative effectiveness.

Such a model may be a practical impossibility, given the history of disagreement in the entire field of community adaptation, especially regarding the factors to be examined when assessing successful adaptation.

While there is no one categorization scheme that exhausts all forms of CRFs, it is clear that many forms do exist. The New Start program, for example, was a "maximum independence" apartment-placement program. It featured: a.) partial staff supervision, b.) resident apartments nested within "normal" apartment complexes, c.) resident responsibility for all personal expenses, and d.) a program of activities and groups that was based upon the principles of normalization, the developmental model, and the doctrine of least restrictive environment. Other kinds of CRFs range from simple board-and- care homes to foster family homes, adult group homes, and mini-institutions.

The labeling of types of CRFs is in itself an activity that reveals the multitude of opinions in the field. There are various categorization schemes based upon differing criteria, in turn yielding different results. Baker, Seltzer, and Seltzer (1977), for instance, have identified 10 classifications of CRFs. They considered three key factors when assigning membership: existing models, facility size, and nature of the program.

Heal et al. (1978) collapsed the Baker et al. list of 10 into four groups with multiple levels. However, Heal et al. found better grouping criteria within the governmental guidelines that regulate these facilities. More recent schema have been proposed by Hill and Lakin (1986). The earlier examples of divergent criteria typify the disagreement, as well as the disorder, prevalent in the field.

Bjaanes and Butler (1974) grouped CRFs according to the degree of normalization programming made available to the residents. They distinguished among custodial, therapeutic, or maintaining facilities. In the custodial site they found that "little or nothing was done to facilitate the normalization process; there was little supervision and only minimal activities for the residents" (p.430). The therapeutic CRF offered a "regular" normalization program, while the maintaining type fell in between, offering more of a program than the custodial but less of a program than the therapeutic types.

Fritz, Wolfensberger, and Knowlton (1971) proposed a subtaxonomy only for apartment placement programs. They described three types: the apartment cluster, the single co-residence apartment with live-in staff, and the maximum independence apartment without live-in staff. They emphasized the level of staff supervision as a key criterion.

As a factor, level of supervision can also be interpreted as an indicator of the level of resident independence. Widespread disagreement within the field on issues such as identification of assessment factors or establishment of generally accepted classification criteria has affected the ability to assess normalization.

Fritz et al. (1971) were among the first to suggest that staff supervision be considered as a key variable. The question of resident independence, how much to allow and when, underlies how much supervision a given CRF decides to provide residents. Until recently, very few programs featured less than total supervision of their residents. Wyngaarden and Gollay (1976) reported that 91.2 percent of the 250 CRFs they surveyed provided around-the-clock staff supervision. Baker, Seltzer, and Seltzer (1974) corroborated this finding, citing less than five percent of their sample as offering less than around-the-clock supervision.

Maximum independence apartment-placement programs, free of 24-hour supervision, are comparatively new. Their divergence from the bulk of CRFs is radical and, to some researchers, confounding. Bruininks (1980), for instance, excluded them entirely from 24-hour, seven-day-a-week CRFs, but at the same time included them with natural family residences and unlicensed board-and-care homes. Clearly, they are vastly different from the latter facilities, often referred to as "flophouses" because of the absence of any program activities.

As a CRF, an apartment-placement program is unique in at least two ways: by design, there is substantially less than around-the-clock supervision; and by intent, the habilitation program adheres to the three principles of normalization, the developmental model, and least restrictive environment.

During the time of this study, Project New Start was considered the vanguard representative of least-restrictive apartment-placement programs. Similar programs existed in the metropolitan area, however, none featured the absence of ongoing, continuous staff supervision that was a central tenet of New Start. Within a few years, however, several new programs emerged that supplanted New Start as the preeminent example of its type.

Although normalization has enjoyed widespread acceptance and has proven to be pivotal in reducing the institutional population by 25 percent, as a national policy it has yet to be adequately evaluated. Zigler's (1976) comment emphasized this point:

> At the social policy level, the mental retardation field is in a state of flux and disarray. Some years ago, experts convinced decision-makers that special education was the solution to the problems of training the retarded. This view is now suspect and decision-makers are now committing themselves to such concepts as normalization and deinstitutionalization. I join with those many senior workers in the field who view these concepts as little more than slogans that are badly in need of an empirical data base.

The evaluation of these programs built on principles such as normalization can provide an empirical data base from which to judge their wisdom. However, there remain obstacles bound in long-standing practices of scientific tradition that inhibit useful evaluation. For example, the single greatest obstacle to effective evaluation has been the failure of researchers to identify salient variables that might describe the process of achieving successful community adaptation.

In the past, these variables have been investigated with the intent to discover their predictive value. Their selection as likely predictors has been, at best, well-intended and, at worst, capricious. They have been investigated as variables belonging to one of two groups: individual traits or programmatic factors. Investigation of variables within each category has relied on the quantitative approach, which is in itself predictive. A careful review of the history of research in this field shows that this search for significant, prognostic variables, both individual-based and program-based, has been uniformly exhaustive, misguided, and fruitless.

The Search for Predictor Variables in Community Adjustment

Goddard (1909) is credited by Eagle (1967) as the first individual to call for the discovery of factors that would forecast the future performance of retarded persons. Goddard felt it would be useful to be able to tell "at the very outset where this child is in mental development and what we may expect from him."

Despite the efforts of many researchers, a system that predicts how a person with mental retardation will adjust to placement in the community does not yet exist. Research has followed a pattern of interest swinging from individual-focused variables (into the 1960s) to program and environment-focused variables (to the present day). When research on individual variables proved fruitless, interest in program variables grew stronger. This pendulum-like pattern of interest roughly coincides with changes over the past half-century in beliefs about people with mental retardation. These beliefs have changed from a "social menace"/alien model to one of "kinship."

The "social menace"/alien model prevailed until the 1960s. Mentally retarded citizens were viewed as radically different human beings, fundamentally distinct from, and perhaps dangerous to, the normal population. Coincidentally, research centered on two similar themes. There were studies of the success/failure rate of institutionalized retardates released into the community. These studies actually grappled with the public's concern for the wisdom of allowing such a potentially hazardous policy to exist. Corollary studies from the same epoch sought to discover the fundamental differences (IQ, age, physical appearance) that would clearly separate people with mental retardation from the rest of humanity.

The "social menace"/alien model was replaced by the "kinship" model. People with mental retardation were now capable of living in the community. They were still imperfect, but no longer considered dangerous. They were even lovable. They were of the same family as normals, but like poor country cousins, they were out of step with the rest of society and in need of training. Research stayed in step. A new generation of studies sought to demonstrate the ability of these individuals to adapt and to adjust to the community.

Eagle (1967) exhaustively documented this resarch. His thorough review made clear some discomforting points. These are that research results could be easily reinterpreted to discredit the policy of institutional release, and that the research in this field has long been characterized by disagreement and futility. His examination of all of the critical studies published over nearly 50 years covered works on individual and program variables. In general, these studies were published during the "social menace" era. Although conclusions about the effects of specific variables were often drawn, they were typically interpolated from frequency data on release rates from and return rates to institutions. They were little more than informed opinions.

Eagle's meta-analysis reviewed a broad sample of investigation from the 1940s through the 1960s, using success and failure as review criteria. His reexamination of 112 studies from 1919 to 1960 (acknowledging Windle, 1962, as his source) and of 36 studies published between 1941 and 1967, presented evidence that the success rates of community programs over the prior half-century actually diminished.

Using Windle's (1962) data, Eagle computed a 27.5 percent failure rate through 1960. Compared with Fernald's 25-year follow-up study in 1919, which found a 36.1 percent failure rate, this finding at first seemed to represent an improvement. However, Eagle showed that a further breakdown of the studies by era suggests that the 41-year failure rate (27.5 percent) is biased by low rates bunched in the earlier years that offset higher rates later on.

For example, the 36 studies from 1941 to 1967 showed a 36.9 percent failure rate. Presuming that "the placement process has benefited within recent years from new developments in the various disciplines involved," Eagle computed a failure rate of 52 percent from the 11 studies conducted between 1960 and 1967 that assessed community placement of the retarded. Eagle's implication—that community placement was not clearly associated with successful adjustment in spite of almost 50 years of effort—was disturbing. But his claim that the failure rate for retarded citizens placed in the community was actually increasing was alarming. The importance of understanding the process of community adjustment for people with mental retardation was bolstered by Eagle's findings.

Eagle also combed the literature on the investigation of predictor variables in community adjustment. The diversity of foci found among researchers was remarkable. The divergence of their results was astounding. For example, sterility of the patient as a predictor variable was investigated by Johnson (1946), Shafter (1957), and Madison (1964). The authors differed and their results were inconclusive. Physical defects as a variable were reported on by Brown (1952), and O'Connor (1957), who found that defects were significant predictors (although others disagreed—see Eagle, 1967, p.237).

At first, studies focusing on individual traits as variables were most favored by researchers. An exception was Shafter (1954), who raised questions about the relative impact certain program variables (such as personnel, selection criteria, and written rules) might have on success. Sarason and Gladwin (1958) were among the earliest to investigate program variables as predictors. They concluded that the criteria typically employed to assess mental deficiency (IQ tests, personality assessments) were inadequate for use as predictors of "social and occupational success or failure."

Macmillan (1962) criticized the focus on individual differences. He suggested that studies interested in prediction of successsful community adjustment had failed because they looked at the wrong set of criteria: IQ, age, physical appearance, and personality. Macmillan proposed that the discharge and adjustment processes themselves be considered for research.

Eagle is the authority for studies on predictor variables published before 1967. He covered research on factors including gender, IQ, length of prior institutionalization, age at institutional release, placement site conditions, religious affiliation, job history, and so forth. His review showed that, in the search for the elusive predictors, the researcher's imagination and perseverance was significant.

Results, unfortunately, remained confusing. As an example, Eagle cited Shafter (1957), who found that release characteristics without prognostic value included emotional dependence on the home, history of sex delinquency, religious affiliation, frequent job changes, gregariousness, neuropathic ancestry, interest in the opposite sex, sibling rank, poorly developed recreational interest, neatness, personal cleanliness, personal appearance, or the ability to read, write, or tell time.

In the same study, Shafter found that positively related variables included truthfulness, ambition, obedience, and good work. Factors that were negatively associated with successful adjustment included aggressiveness, carelessness, history of institutional escape, history of stealing, quarrelsomeness, and having been "excessively punished."

Eagle (1967) found that the reasons most often cited in the literature for explaining failure fell into the following categories; antisocial problems, undesirable personal conduct, personal problems, unsatisfactory work habits, health problems, escape or voluntary return to the institution, adverse environmental factors, and transfer to another facility. Eagle closed his epic review succinctly:

> Published data on more than 30 release characteristics for their prognostic value for success or non-success in community placement of previously institutionalized retardates showed wide disagreement as to their utility (1967, p.241).

Research on Individual-Focused Variables

This body of literature also has a long-standing history. Only recently has a body of work begun to emerge that examines the relationship between individual traits, especially those that are psychologically related, and adjustment as a little understood phenomenon rather than as a predictor. Examples of this new direction include investigations by Levine (1985) in his work on "situational" (i.e., performance) anxiety; Linden and Forness (1986) on the effects of a "dual-diagnosis" (mental retardation and mentally disordered) on community adjustment; and Matson (1984) on the need for and benefit of supportive psychotherapy for mildly mentally retarded persons placed in the community.

This literature is more typically represented by the work of Brown, Windle, and Stewart (1959), who wrote that "the most frequent reasons for rehospitalization involve conditions of the patient. . .(p.538)." Windle, Stewart, and Brown (1961) found that the chief reasons for community adjustment failure as cited in ten key studies could be grouped under two headings: personal behavior (*antisocial, intolerable*) or personality traits (*character defects, personality factors*).

Beliefs based in fear about people with mental retardation spurred individual-focused research. Kernan, Turner, Langness, and Edgerton (1978) documented the extreme biases that have influenced research in mental retardation, especially as it pertains to community placement and adjustment. They listed sample beliefs "supported" by research:

1. The mentally retarded have a significantly higher incidence of personality disorder than comparable normal populations (Beier, 1964; Garrison & Force, 1965; Hirsch, 1959; Hutt & Gibby, 1965; Johnson, 1963).
2. Certain personality characteristics (e.g., rigidity, anxiety, suggestibility, "ego limitation," etc.) are concommitant with intellectual retardation (Feldman, 1946; Hirsch, 1959; Lewin, 1936).
3. Certain personality traits are predictive of success and failure in postinstitutional adjustment (Cobb, 1923; McPherson, 1935; Windle, 1962). (Kernan et al., 1978, pp.18-19).

The need to isolate people with retardation from the community was a great one. Beliefs reinforced by research provided ample justification. However, as Eagle found, the overall body of research did not provide conclusive evidence to support the beliefs. In fact, conclusions drawn by many of the investigators ultimately discredited the value of individual traits as significant variables.

Windle et al. (1961) noted that the most frequently cited reason for placement failure after personal behavior and personality factors was poor health and lack of environmental support. They suggested that differences observed between success and failure of released patients might not be a result of personal factors alone. "Large differences among patients released on different types of leave. . . (suggest) that different processes leading to reinstitutionalization take place in different programs (p.217)."

Windle was one of the most active researchers of individual-focused variables, yet he felt that a nonindividual variable (differences between programs) might also play an important role. Similar ambivalence about one's own conclusions is found in the work of Windle's colleagues as well.

Sternlicht (1978) listed four sources of variables that "influence the probability of successful foster care placement for retarded individuals discharged into the community" (p.25). They are the resident, the foster parents or caretakers, the community, and the institution. Although Sternlicht listed four sources, he devoted the great bulk of his attention to one: the resident/individual. His literature review confirms that the majority of research on community adjustment has focused on the "unique" personal characteristics of the individual with retardation.

Sternlicht found that unacceptable behavior was "of paramount importance in successful placements"; that poor health, corroborated by his own research, was important; that researchers disagreed about the significance of the resident's age; that mild to moderately retarded individuals are more at risk than those with lower IQ levels (again corroborated by his own research); that gender is an inconsistent predictor; and, finally, that independence in self-care is more significant than other skill factors.

Taylor (1976) found that the adaptive behaviors most troublesome for residents in group homes, resulting in their return to the institution, were untrustworthy behavior, poor money management, poor number and time concepts, and hyperactivity. On the other hand, behaviors that Taylor found to be tolerated in the homes included inappropriate personal manners, psychological disturbances, and rebelliousness.

Hull and Thompson (1980) examined variables of individuals and residences and concluded that a "variety of individual characteristics, especially IQ, are related to adaptive functioning" (p.259). Other noteworthy variables included age and behavior problems. Hull and Thompson interpreted their results with an underlying sense of futility. They felt that finding individual characteristics to be among the stronger determinants of successful community adjustment proved of questionable utility. They pointed out that findings of this sort "offer little hope to planners who wish to improve the adaptive functioning level of retarded persons as these characteristics are either extremely difficult and costly to change, if they can be changed at all—IQ, behavioral problems, or impossible to change—age" (1980, p.259).

Unlike Hull and Thompson, investigators McCarver and Craig (1973), along with Aininger and Bolinsky (1977), found that IQ was related to successful adjustment. Sutter, Mayeda, Call, Yanagi, and Yee (1980) found that more females were successful than males in community placement but, they added, this is inconsistent with the research of Brown (1952), who found males more successful, and Tarjan, Dingman, Eyman, and Brown (1959), who found gender and placement failure unrelated.

Sutter et al. also found residents with lower IQs to be less successful than residents with higher IQs. These findings countered those of Morissey (1966), where higher IQs were more successful, but corroborated Bishop (1957), and Windle, Stewart, and Brown (1961). Tarjan found no connection between IQ and successful community placement. More recently, King, Soucer, and Isset (1980) found that none of the four most popular predictor variables (gender, age at admission, IQ, and etiological diagnosis) discriminated among groups.

Extensive research on individual-focused variables has ultimately demonstrated the lack of value they hold as revealing phenomena. Edgerton and Bercovici (1976) may have understated this when they wrote that "there is a large literature in which it is consistently reported that the best available prognostic variables, whether measures of attitude, personality skills, or life circumstances, have failed to be accurate predictors of community adjustment" (p.489).

Research on Program (Environmental)-Focused Variables

The shift in focus on research from individual to program variables happened slowly. Issues of methodology as well as variable selection came under scrutiny in the transition. Early studies sometimes advised that research on placement success should include research on the placement programs themselves.

Brown, Windle, and Stewart (1959) called for more investigations of "a.) the effects of various types of family care programs, and b.) prognostic factors for each type of program" (p.542). More recently, Bjaanes and Butler (1974) presented a brief but informative review describing environmental effects as being multileveled, and directly related to successful community adjustment. They cited studies on the "positive" effect, which change in setting (PRF to CRF) had on IQ levels (McKay, 1942; Mundy, 1957; Skeels & Dye, 1939) as well as social and verbal behavior (Tizard, 1960). They also cited Edgerton (1967) and Dingman (1967) as having been among the first to suggest that the process of community adjustment cannot be completely understood without knowledge of the setting in which it occurs.

Using a modified participant observation model, Bjaanes and Butler (1974) made comparisons across types of facilities. They hoped to break ground in the development of an overall evaluation model. They observed "substantial differences. . .in the environment of community care facilities" (p.438) and concluded that "the development of independent functioning and social competence appears to be related to geographical location of the facility, and involvement of the caretaker" (p.439).

Furthermore, "specific types of community care environments are associated with different outcomes" (p.439). They carefully cautioned the reader to consider their findings as "tentative and explanatory" because of the small sample size and "all the vagaries and difficulties inherent in the development and testing of a new research design" (p.439).

Bjaanes and Butler's tentativeness can be attributed to the newness of the territory they felt they were entering. Their caution also can be seen as endemic of the vagueness encountered by most of the researchers who began investigating program/environmental variables. This quickly proved to be a task of greater complexity than investigation of individual variables. Multiple domains of variables (program operations, staff, physical plant, etc.) confronted researchers where only one domain (the individual) had before. Program-variable researchers were confounded not only by the unclear boundaries of their investigations but also by the emerging question of methodological appropriateness.

Bjaanes and Butler were among the earliest to attempt the use of nonquantitative methods where quantitative procedures had always been the previous method of choice. The earliest studies on individual variables had dealt almost exclusively with archival frequency data (length of stay, age, test scores, etc.). Programmatic and environmental data proved more difficult to quantify. Researchers apparently preferred working with numerical data. It seems that they looked for the variables that were most easily quantified, taking a stab-in-the-dark approach to variable selection. These variables were analyzed and reanalyzed until they proved profitless. One legacy of this approach is the body of research on the possible relationship of size of facilities to successful adaptation. Bercovici (1978) comments on this point:

> The assumption that 'big is bad' and the expectation that removal of the mentally retarded to a smaller residential setting would ameliorate the effects of institutionalization have not been borne out...the emphasis on the variable of size has been shown to be an inadequate conceptualization of the problem" (p.3).

Balla (1976) reviewed this same literature and, in words kinder than Bercovici's but no less discouraging, concluded:

> ...there is little evidence to suggest that the behavioral functioning of residents is different in institutions of different sizes. There are essentially no data on the issue of whether smaller institutions are more adequate than larger ones in terms of returning their residents to the community" (p.122).

Difficulty in conceptualizing the problem of measuring and targeting influences appears with regularity in this literature. In fact, it becomes apparent that the problems of targeting program/environmental variables and measuring them are closely intertwined. Many studies have unintentionally revealed the incongruity of doing environmental research via experimental methods.

Pratt, Luszcz, and Brown (1980), in an attempt to develop "tools for the measurement of care across a variety of residential settings," tried adapting four measurement scales used in evaluating large institutions to an evaluation of the quality of care in small, community-based group homes. They concluded that their adaptation proved reliable and valid in the strictest measurement sense, but they remained reluctant to draw any conclusions about the quality of care (p.193). Their use of strict measurement technique in this case was not helpful.

Aininger and Bolinsky (1977) wanted to examine placement success in an apartment-living program. They analysed pre and post scores on behavior rating scales. They also factor-analyzed individual traits such as IQ, examining strength of association traits and rating scale scores. They intended to assess whether the move from "formal institution living to a more independent living situation (was) a stepping stone to independence or...a good alternative to deinstitutionalization" (p.12). Their study, however, is cited most often for its contribution in linking IQ and adjustment, not independent living and independence. The tendency to look at such research in terms that are familiar (correlations) rather than novel is almost automatic, despite intentions to the contrary.

Eyman, Demaine, and Lei (1979) investigated an apparent misconception in the evaluation of normalization programs. Quoting Meisbou (1976), they observed that the primary normalization evaluation tool, the PASS (Program

Analysis of Service Systems), measures the conformity of service systems to the normalization principle, "whereas the real issue should be the effect of these systems on the individuals they are designed to serve" (p.331). They were attempting a new approach, hoping to uncover new information about the program and its participants. They factor-analyzed PASS and the AAMR Adaptive Behavior Scale scores, associating them with individual variables (age, IQ, and initial adaptive behavior level). Their study of "community environments and adaptive behavior" found that "older, less retarded residents improved in overall adaptive behavior regardless of where they reside." Their results were neither new nor conclusive, being in agreement with Morrissey (1966), but in opposition to Bishop (1957), Windle et al. (1961), and Sutter et al. (1980).

Researchers have seemingly exhausted the universe of variables that might in some combination successfully predict community adaptation of persons with mental retardation. Despite these efforts, understanding of community adaptation has not been enhanced. Methodological possibilities, however, have not been exhausted. Two basic methodologies have dominated the literature, with one far outstripping the other in frequency of appearance. They are archival analyses (i.e., the examination of existing records) and quasi-experimental designs with quantitative statistical analyses on scores from behavior rating scales. Very few studies have employed qualitative methods of any sort.

Related Recent Research on the Role of Friendship in Community Adaptation

In 1979 Landesman-Dwyer, Berkson, and Romer published one of the first articles to focus on friendship as a factor in the adaptation of people with mental retardation. The literature on the importance of friendship to adaptation is, in general, relatively broad and often found in loosely related areas. Heller, Rasmussen, Cook, and Wolosin (1981), for example, investigated the relationship between neighborhood strain resulting from changing community composition and its effect on residents' satisfaction. Among their conclusions was that "satisfaction was most closely linked to personal and neighborhood ties. Friends in the neighborhood and a spouse who is available as a companion were the best predictors of neighborhood satisfaction" (p.41).

Procidano and Heller (1983) reviewed three studies addressing the belief that personal needs for social support are being adequately met (i.e., perceived social support, or PSS). In their article, the authors distinguished between social networks and social support, describing the former as the "social connections provided by the environment" and the latter as the "impact networks have on the individual."

They further distinguished between PSS Fr (from friends) and PSS Fa (from family) stating that "the distinction between friend support and family support is considered important . . . (as) Different populations . . . may rely on or benefit from friend or family support to different extents" (p.2). They further suggested that social competence weighs heavily in the maintenance of a support network, especially if that network is based in friendship rather than family. The implications for adaptation of people with mild mental retardation should be obvious. Programs should assess the extent and nature of each participant's social network.

Furthermore, these networks should be featured in the Individual Program Plan as necessary resources for promoting and managing independent living. In the absence of social networks, the creation of a network for each individual should be paramount if the expectation of successful independent living is to be realized.

Heller had the opportunity to apply his findings on the importance of friendship networks to well-being (a suicide prevention strategy) as described in an article by Fondacaro, Heller, and Reilly (1984). This unusual convergence of theory and practice occurred in response to a rash of suicidal gestures in a large, high-rise, on-campus dormitory for graduate students. In an effort to "reduce feelings of loneliness and to increase social interaction among residents" the authors proposed a program to develop social networks in the dormitory. After one year of workshops and seminars, the authors cautiously reported that the incidence of suicidal gestures vanished.

Boruchow and Espenshade (1976) described a program for enhancing the socialization skills of young retarded adults through low-key group therapies. While the program described was very simple in conception, it nevertheless offered recognition for the importance of social skills in achieving independent living.

Seltzer (1985) described the compensatory benefits of informal support networks of family and friends on aging people with mental retardation. Stainback and Stainback (1987) proposed a model for teaching people with mental retardation how to make and retain friends using a technique they referred to as *coaching*.

In the same article, the authors upgraded social skills to friendship skills, with specific descriptions. Finally, Rhoades, Browning, and Thorin (1986) lobbied for adoption of peer-support systems in the form of self-help advocacy groups as an integral part of independent living programs. Participation in self-help groups, they argued, improved the identity of persons with mental retardation as well as affording them the opportunity to develop meaningful friendships with peers.

In their article, Rhoades et al. presented many of the concerns that are often voiced as obstructions to the development of friendships among the retarded, including the stigma of being labeled, or of associating with those who are labeled.

The literature on the friendships of people with mental retardation is limited. It is further constrained by the point of view commonly underlying published studies: the inherent assumption that more contact with family and friendship networks is intrinsically beneficial. This bias is so prevalent that it leaves the reader with the impression that life is truly like the song "You Gotta Have Friends."

Zetlin and Turner (1985) provided one of the rare alternative perspectives that such is not always the case.

For example, they wrote that "(Parents) are more likely to encourage dependency, obedience and child-like behavior than independence, self-direction, assumption of responsibility and sexual awareness" (p.571).

In describing their sample of 46 retarded adults and their networks of family and friends, they concluded that three classifications of adaptive styles emerged: independent adults were those individuals who "handled most of the everyday affairs of their lives without assistance and only in times of crisis turned to parents for support"; dependent adults "looked to their parents for protection and guidance in virtually every dimension of their lives"; and interdependent adults who were "enmeshed in conflict-ridden relationships with parents." This last group "solicited extensive assistance but resented accompanying attempts by parents to exert control over their activities. Parents preferred less involvement but insisted on maintaining control over decisions affecting their child's life. These were the least well adjusted members of the sample" (p.578).

Zetlin and Turner's portrayal of adjustment issues during retarded persons' adolescence, and the subsequent effects on their adult lives, dissents from the more simplistic formula often found in more current advocacy tomes.

Methodology and the Study of Community Adjustment

The early studies published through the 1950s relied almost exclusively on archival data. Landmark works such as those by Fernald (1919), Brown, Windle, and Stewart (1959), and Windle, Stewart, and Brown (1961), for example, used institutional records of former and current residents as data sources. Descriptive statistics were reported.

The presence of people with mental retardation in the community always seems to have been meticulously reported, creating an abundance of frequency data. Quasi-experimental designs permitting the use of powerful statistical analyses on these data presently dominate the literature. Techniques that have been employed to analyze the data have varied widely, including multivariate analysis (Aininger & Bolinsky, 1977; Baldwin, 1978; Taylor, 1976), multiple regression (Hull & Thompson, 1980), discriminant function analysis and simple t-test (King et al., 1980). Sutter et al. (1980) used nonparametric statistics to analyze differences between scores on behavior ratings. Some researchers have supplemented their quasi-experimental models with qualitative techniques in the data gathering. Such studies, which have employed structured interviews and limited participant observations, have been assessed by Gollay (1976), and Aininger and Bolinsky (1977).

The number of studies relying primarily on qualitative methods is minimal. Those that do employ these methods do so marginally and, as a result, fail to take advantage of the methods' powers. Crnic and Pym (1979), for instance, had program staff act as participant observers, rating residents' skill levels on five-point scales. Simple means were reported. Bjaanes and Butler (1974) used a modified participant observation model to generate frequencies of behavioral data (relationship and social skills). They analyzed the expected frequencies by chi-square and reported simple differences between intact groups, nothing more.

Apart from this group are the researchers who have utilized qualitative methods in more conventional forms. Bercovici (1981, 1983), Edgerton (1967, 1977, 1988), Edgerton and Bercovici (1976), Levine (1981, 1985), Levine and Langness (1985), Sullivan, Vitello, and Foster (1988), and Zetlin and Turner (1985) represent a group of investigators who have successfully employed a radically different approach to research in this field. They have drawn directly from the tradition of ethnography and phenomenology.

From numerous standpoints this tradition is the polar opposite of quantitative methods. Quantitative methods are based in the positivist tradition, which seeks to discover laws by which phenomena can be predicted. The phenomenology approach, on the other hand, seeks understanding. This understanding derives not only from the participant's perspective but also from his experience, part of which the researcher might in some way share (Smith, 1983). In the search for variables adequate to describe successful community adaptation, the use of qualitative methods is indicated, if for no other reason than the complete failure of quantitative methods to accomplish the task. Qualitative methods offer certain features that seem uniquely suited to the study of community adaptation. These features are discussed in the next section.

The Development and Use of Qualitative Methods in Evaluation

The field of evaluation has emerged by necessity—the result of applying a political solution to a social problem. Patton (1978) traced the roots of evaluation to the Great Depression and New Deal eras, when straightforward program histories were regularly collected on the numerous public programs of the time. He identified the political and social turmoil of the 1960s and 1970s as the blast furnaces that helped forge the "industry" of evaluation as we know it today:

"It was not until the massive federal expenditures on an awesome assortment of programs during the 1960's and 1970's that accountability began to mean more than assessing staff sincerity or political headcounts of opponents and proponents...These Great Society programs collided head-on with the Vietnam War, rising inflation, increasing taxes, and the fall from glory of Keynesian economics...From all the turmoil of that period, something called 'evaluation research' emerged as an alternative. . .to assessing program effectiveness. By the early 1970's evaluations were being regularly required of health, education, and welfare programs (Patton, 1978, pp.14, 15).

At first, the demand for program evaluation easily exceeded the development of evaluation technology. The field was in its infancy without benefit of parentage. There was no heritage from which to draw. Methodology and theory had to be developed immediately, or adopted in the meantime from a related field. Quantitative methods and experimental theory provided a solution. The early misnomer "evaluation research" reflected this initial marriage between evaluation and quantitative methods.

Weiss (1970) was a prominent advocate for "good" evaluations, which, in her opinion, observed the basic canons of "good" research—that is, the use of control groups and sound statistical methods to ensure reliability and validity of results. Rossi, Freeman, and Wright (1979) formalized this position. They advocated "systematic evaluations" with "distinguishing characteristics," which was simply another euphemism for experimental tenets. "Distinguishing characteristics" were a.) observations that could be "duplicated by others using the same instruments" (replicability), and b.) "evidence of results proven by tests which show that the findings would not occur without the intervention" (control groups).

The alignment of evaluation with qualitative models in social science research provided an initial sense of legitimacy and maturity to the fledgling field. In time, however, evaluators increasingly voiced dissatisfaction that their evaluation results were not being utilized (Alkin, 1981; Patton, 1978, Weiss, 1972). Explanations of nonutilization were sought, such as concern for the evaluator's proper role (Alkin, 1978; Scriven, 1973; Stake, 1972). Along with other concerns to be discussed below, this opened up the field to consideration of other methodological alternatives.

Scriven (1973) stated that the evaluator should look for any and all effects of a given program rather than enter the evaluation with preconceived notions as to what comprises success or failure. He called this approach *goal-free evaluation*. Paying attention to stated program goals biased the evaluator unfavorably, compromising his role. Scriven questioned the language of quantitative methods, particularly standard references to unanticipated findings as "side effects," "secondary effects," or "unanticipated effects." He suggested it might be best for the evaluator not to anticipate any effects so as best to evaluate all effects.

Stake (1972) addressed the same family of issues with his Responsive Evaluation model, which sought to effect a "natural fit" with the existing program structure. He argued that this was preferable to forcing an experimental model upon an already loose and hard-to-systematize world of experience. Stake felt that evaluation should respond to the audience's requirements for information, represent the audience's perspectives, and be oriented to program process rather than program intent. This model was an alternative to what he termed *Preordinate Evaluation,* which a.) assumed a statement of goals (hypotheses), b.) used objective tests to collect data (nonparticipatory), c.) followed the programs' directions for program assessment (constraint of assumptions), and d.) resulted in a research-type report. Stake (1978) also argued for the usefulness of the case study method as an appropriate evaluation model. He defended this method against criticisms commonly made of qualitative methods.

For example, in response to the contention that qualitative methods are not replicable and therefore not open to generalization, he suggested that these concepts be reconsidered in actual evaluation-practice terms. In evaluation, he argued, one needs "particular case generalization," as opposed to population-wide generalization. Evaluations, he proposed, served narrow situations, not broad ones. The aim was therefore to make one's special case recognizable through excellence of description.

Eisner (1981) continued to articulate the differences between qualitative and quantitative methods as applied to evaluation. He distinguished between the scientific and artistic approaches to research. In artistic research standardized tests would not be the instrument of choice because they insulated the investigator from the business of data collection. For the artistic researcher, personal experience of the setting was critical. For the scientist, it was irrelevant. While the scientist searched for "truth," the artist searched for "understanding."

Eisner's observations were not isolated musings. Presented less poetically but no less emphatically were the sympathetic thoughts of Guba (1978). "Useful evaluation information is not often produced (and) a major reason seems to be lack of a methodology uniquely suited to evaluation's needs" (p.1). Furthermore, Guba cited Scriven (1972), Cronbach (1975), and Tymitz and Wolf (1977) as being among those evaluators who, like himself, disagreed with the suggestion that qualitative methods are less scientific than quantitative methods.

Qualitative methods are theory or question generating. New questions are answered only to discover newer ones. It is an expansive model of inquiry that depends on richness and rigor of description to ensure that data are both reliable and valid.

Today, widespread support for qualitative methods can be found in the literature of educational research. Gage (1989) summarized the paradigms as those of interpretivists and criticalists, while burying the hatchet on the controversy by acknowledging that both positions have their place in research.

The mental retardation literature, by contrast, has not been swept along in the tide of richer description. Very few apartment-placement program evaluations can be found that employ naturalistic techniques. It should be noted that two earlier studies (Aininger & Bolinsky, 1977; Baldwin, 1978) were neither "true" evaluations nor strong examples of naturalistic reporting. They did not document the experiences of the participants from an emic (insiders') perspective. Although the Aininger and Bolinsky (1977) study used qualitative methods (participant observation) in the data collection and triangulation of data sources to ensure validity, virtually no description of the program or the participants was provided. Neither the Aininger and Bolinsky study nor the Baldwin study presented a description of the program from the participants' view. This tendency was often found in the research on community adjustment programs, and was decried by Bercovici (1981):

> Among all the finely honed research that has been done in the area of community placement, the writer has yet to see a complete description of even one residential facility and the daily life of its residents. . .While this is not a critique of quantitative methodologies, it is a suggestion that researchers might be using their techniques too exclusively in attempting to understand and describe what is a complex situation of social change" (p.134).

Chapter 3

Description of the Program, the Sample, and the Research Procedures

Description of Project New Start

Project New Start was founded in 1976. Two former employees wrote the following succinct description of the program in 1983:

> New Start (was an) independent living program with three sites in the Los Angeles area. Project New Start is one of the programs under the umbrella agency called HOK, Help Our Kids. HOK was organized approximately nine years ago by parents of developmentally disabled adults seeking out services for their children. Project New Start was designed to educate adults with special needs in areas of basic independent living skills and vocational education. The program refers to its developmentally disabled clients as tenants...Tenants live in apartments in the community near the individual office sites. They each live with a roommate and each pair of roommates is responsible for paying all bills and maintaining the apartment. Tenants are expected to participate in a daily activity apart from a Project New Start sponsored program. The average length-of-stay is approximately two years. The ultimate goal upon completion is for tenants to live independently and be competitively employed. Project New Start's clients consist of individuals who have either cerebral palsy, epilepsy, are mildly mentally retarded, or a combination of these (Hutchisson & Rush, 1983).

More than 300 adults with developmental disabilities had successfully applied and enrolled in the program since its inception in 1976. Once admitted, they were eligible for two immediate program benefits: assignment to a program-sponsored apartment which they shared with another participant; and assignment to a counselor, who was responsible for helping develop a weekly schedule of activities along with preparing the individual program plan complete with personal goals.

Activities were typically separated into those for daytime (e.g., workshop, job, psychotherapy), and those for evening (e.g., social, group and individual instruction). This schedule changed periodically as participants moved through various program stages. Graduation to independent living status was the overall goal. The program sought to follow participants through periodic social or instructional contacts for a period of time after graduation.

Training in independent living skills, as conducted by the counselors, occurred either during daytime or evening activities. This training covered the traditional areas of money management, housekeeping, food preparation, grocery shopping, banking, and public transportation. Langone and Burton (1987) have neatly dissected the array of skills common to the training of people with retardation into categories which merit mention. Their categories include skills generally found in this type of program as well as some not so common. These are self-care, home management, consumer behaviors, and community mobility. While Langone and Burton's intentions seem to have been simply to provide a sensible, well-organized taxonomy of skills, they also performed a service to the entire field by cogently discriminating among levels of skills which all too often are lumped under the broad heading of independent living.

New Start counselors carried a caseload of participants with whom they were responsible to meet several times per week. During these meetings they were to provide assistance in basic living skills, conduct informal counseling, note any significant changes such as progress in the individual program plan, etc. The balance of time not spent with residents was for charting and staff meetings. While the job did not seem to be demanding on paper, there was evidence that program staff often felt incompetent or ill prepared for their task.

Because program participants were supposed to have already mastered the basic living skills, counselors were informed that they would be providing only supplementary support in these areas. In fact, several of the counselors interviewed commented on their lack of preparation and training in these areas.

A study by Slater and Bunyard (1983) described how frequently this sort of complaint was found among program staff. In their study of 92 CRF staff members from Wisconsin they found that less than 50 percent could correctly identify basic social training tools such as modeling, praise, or punishment. Despite this, between 75 and 85 percent identified communication skills, independent living skills, socialization, and emotional development as essential participant needs.

New Start also offered a social skills program in which the counselors found it equally difficult to feel and act like experts. Counselors were encouraged to organize ongoing support groups among program participants residing in the same apartment complex. The purpose of these meetings was not always apparent. They were not necessarily oriented toward the development of friendship skills, at least as described in other research on modeling groups by Stainback and Stainback (1987). These two investigators have argued that friendship is a complex matter essential to social, emotional, and physical health and well-being. As such, friendship could be task analyzed, defined differentially from social interaction and popularity, and taught via a process they refer to as *coaching*. Furthermore, they advocated that coaching should occur in a natural setting allowing for the practice, generalization, and maintenance of friendship skills.

Little of this seemed to have occurred at New Start, due in large part to the counselors' lack of knowledge, the absence of adequate supervision and training, and the program's failure to make friendship a prominent issue, at least not to the same degree reflected in recent research (Stainback & Stainback, 1987; Rhoades, Browning, & Thorin, 1986; Seltzer, 1985; Zetlin & Turner, 1985; Fondacaro, Heller, & Reilly, 1984).

Parental involvement, another important program component, did not appear to be any more effectively or concretely implemented than the social skills/friendship component. Boruchow and Espenshade (1976) described how parents were involved in an independent living skills training program that utilized a quasi-psychotherapy group to compensate for participants' "inadequate socialization" (defined as the *lack of opportunity* to maximize skills inherent to self-care, social interaction, travel and employment).

This program provided group therapy led by a psychologist and a social worker for the participants, along with a parents' group, home visits, and family meetings. Parents and other family members were specifically included. They considered work with the family and all parents to be central to the success of the program. At New Start, the parents (or primary caretakers) were included in the initial assessment of participant's skills. Following that, their ongoing participation was elective and not considered to be central to the New Start program. In some cases the program/family relationship was openly hostile, as naive staff openly clashed with parents over "control" of the participants.

For example, one New Start counselor, promoted from the clerical staff, recounted an incident in which she "proved a point" to her client and the parents. She discovered that one of her clients had been using an elaborate scheme to conceal money spent on prohibited fast food and candy by collecting receipts at markets to represent phony approved expenditures. Earlier the counselor had argued with the parents when she first suspected the scheme. They denied complicity and admonished her suspiciousness. When she confronted the client's parents with the hard evidence, she did so with some pleasure. The ensuing argument escalated to the point that the local New Start administrator had to intervene. This unproductive episode is described in more detail in Chapter 7.

Counselors not only felt as if they were unqualified as counselors and instructors, but also sometimes behaved so. One of the most embarrassing situations for New Start involved a counselor who was released from his position following more than six months of increasingly bizarre behavior. When the counselor initially moved into the same apartment complex where program participants lived, he explained it as a matter of dedication meeting convenience. When other staff verified residents' reports that his apartment was absurdly unkempt, and when he failed to show up for work at regularly scheduled hours (contending that he was performing his duties during more convenient hours) it became clear that he had slowly deteriorated beyond a state which the program could tolerate.

It is not surprising given the ongoing level of confusion among staff members (the preceding two cases illustrating the point) that the turnover rate at New Start steadily escalated so that within four years the average length-of-stay for staff had been halved (see Table 1). Such an outcome would have been difficult for New Start's founding director to reconcile, as he was regarded as an individual whose personal charisma was strong enough to retain a loyal and dedicated (if marginally qualified) staff.

New Start was directed by one person, Darren Mickelson*, during its first seven years of existence. He came to New Start with an MSW degree and previous experience with the Salvation Army as a program developer. During his tenure, the agency demonstrated impressive growth and became known as the most highly regarded program of its kind.

From 1983 through 1984, Project New Start seemed to be at its peak. The programs at all three sites were in great demand. Staff sizes were the largest in program history. Applications and referrals increased so quickly that waiting lists were necessary. According to a New Start senior counselor, the program "used to take everybody, primarily due to money considerations. Now, we have an extensive waiting list for people to come into the program."

New Start's success was relatively short-lived. By 1986 two of the sites had closed, and in early 1987 the program was bankrupt. The New Start program officially operated for 10 years, but functioned as a viable program for only six years (1979 to 1985). A lifetime of five years is not atypical for a semi-independent living program. Hill et al. (1986) reported that "semi-independent living programs were the least stable type of residential placement (programs), with only 40 percent remaining open at the same address over five years."

There were internal circumstances that may have hastened the program's decline. These internal conditions were suggested through discussions with two New Start counselors, one New Start site director, one HOK director, the HOK program evaluator, and a referral agency counselor who had been extensively involved with New Start since 1978. These informants were not representative of all agency staff nor of all peripherally involved professionals. However, their comments and opinions offered a cross-section of personal experiences with New Start during its heyday.

Several external events were suggested by informants as also having contributed to the program's deterioration. For example, state legislation, proposed in early 1984, limited the length of time in which a program participant could enroll in such a program. Also, by 1985 a competitor program had supplanted New Start as the program of choice among counselors at the primary referring agency, the State Disabilities Department (SDD).

The SDD operates offices across the state that register, evaluate, and provide services for all handicapped people, including those with mental retardation. An SDD source commented that, "there was simply too much change

---

*All names used in this manuscript are pseudonyms.

going on (at New Start). We felt disillusioned. The staff turnover was a big problem. I think the quality of counselors changed significantly."

Four internal conditions may have contributed to the decline of Project New Start, but they may also have had implications for the eventual success of program participants. These conditions reflect basic areas of program practice and policy typically of concern to similar organizations or programs. These were a.) staff turnover, b.) program evaluation policy, c.) staff supervision practices, and d.) the role and effect of a prominent leader in the program's development.

Staff Turnover

It is argued that staff turnover is a measure of a program's well-being that is in turn affected by evaluation policy, supervision practices, and leadership. In the case of New Start, staff turnover provided a concrete indicator of the program's relative stability over its lifetime. Program stability as an organizational phenomenon has been examined by others in terms of employee turnover.

Fimian (1983, 1984) applied findings on the determinants of employee turnover in organizational and administrative research to persons who work with the retarded. He investigated the presence of work stress, burnout, needs deficiencies, role conflict, and role ambiguity on personnel employed by community-based programs providing services to adults with mental retardation. He found that the presence of these factors "could result in worker dissatisfaction, contribute to a deteriorating work climate, increase staff turnover rates, and reduce the overall quality of the staff's on-the-job performance."

Bruininks, Kudla, Wieck, and Hauber (1980) found in a national survey of 2,000 CRF administrators that staff turnover was the second most frequently identified problem (first was a lack of qualified staff).

Table 1 below presents data for 91 clinical and administrative staff (excluding clerks) who worked at New Start from 1976 through April 1984 (31 of these individuals were still employed as of April 1984). As can be seen, there was a high incidence as well as an increasing rate of staff turnover. These data suggest that the New Start staff, and consequently the program and participants, probably suffered from Fimian's constellation of problems.

TABLE 1

Staff Turnover at New Start

	1976-1978	1979	1980	1981	1982	1983-1984*
Total Positions	9	16	17	25	31	33
Total Terminated	2	2	9	14	11	22
Total Hired	9	9	10	22	16	23
Current	1	1	1	5	5	18
Avg Months Worked	26.4	22.1	16.8	18.4	13.5	6.9

*Note: Only covers the 16-month period January 1983–April 1984.

The years 1976-1978 and 1983-1984 were collapsed for simplicity. Two staff people, the director and the evaluator who worked there from the beginning, were treated as outliers and excluded from the computation of average months employed.

The average number of months worked decreased significantly between 1979 and 1980, and then again between 1981 and 1982. Almost one-third of the staff hired in 1983 had already departed by early 1984. Employees left in greater numbers and were employed by New Start for briefer lengths of time. Despite the accelerating turnover rate, new staff positions were created routinely. Informants suggested that chronically low pay, difficult working conditions, poor staff training and supervision, an absence of staff material resources, and an apparent lack of a cogent hiring policy contributed to staff turnover. Almost all of these problems were cited by Halpern et al. (1986) as epidemic among semi-independent living programs.

Data for 62 employees who left New Start as of April 1984 were collected from agency records. Reasons for leaving included: returned to school; moved to a better position within the same or a different field; burned out; and fired or left the field. A small percentage of these employees identified other reasons (e.g., moved to state of origin, pregnancy). Table 2 contains data on staff departures for the period 1976 through April 1984.

TABLE 2

Staff Terminations by Reason

	Returned to School	Better Job	Fired/ Burned out	Left Field	Other
Total	8	12*/3**	17	12	8
Percent	13.3%	25%	28.3%	20%	13.3%

*same field
**different field

Nearly half of the 60 employees (17+12=29, 48.3%) left their jobs under duress—they were either fired, burned out, or abandoned the field entirely. On the other hand, relatively few employees (8, or 13.3%) left New Start to return to school. Several agency informants stated that New Start expected staff to use the agency as a stepping stone into the profession of human services. This unofficial yet prevalent policy was apparently intended to encourage staff careerism. Only one third of all terminated employees (8+12=20) returned to school or moved to better jobs in the field, reducing the policy to rhetoric.

Program Evaluation Policy

The task of designing and implementing an agency-wide evaluation strategy was left to one individual, Kay Dooley. She was trained as a social worker and had an extensive background in mental retardation and special programs. As the program evaluator, Dooley described her job as accounting for participant progress and counselor contacts. She adapted the so-called "Blue Form," the program's entry screening device, from existing instruments commonly used by CRFs. Counselors were required to complete the lengthy instrument quarterly. The Blue Form was also New Start's primary program evaluation instrument. It was subsequently used as an exit assessment instrument as well. New Start policy required that clients be rated at a minimum level of performance on all major skills in order to graduate.

The instrument was 24 pages long and contained more than 200 items. Subjects were placed at one of three functional levels on each skill. It was assumed that levels were roughly stable or equivalent across each skill area. However, examination of the items suggested this was not the case. For example, the skills required for level-one hair brushing and level-one money changing were not parallel. Not choosing or not knowing how to brush one's hair did not necessarily explain the same cognitive or cultural deficiencies that pertain to not recognizing or using monetary denominations.

A second component of the program evaluation policy was an attempt to track the program's graduates. By tracking graduates, New Start intended to demonstrate program effectiveness as well as to identify program weaknesses from the planned analysis of completed survey instruments. Dooley, asked to devise a suitable instrument, developed the "Follow-up Form." Inspired by the "Blue Form," it shared the same reductionistic approach to task mastery, also assuming that competency in the tasks measured was important to independent living.

Items on the 12-page form covered eight general areas. Four of these areas drew from core curricula (money management, meal preparation and cooking, personal management, and household maintenance) offered in the New Start program. The remaining four areas (leisure, friendship and dating, use of community resources, and vocation) corresponded to extra-curricular program emphases.

The instrument contained both questions and descriptors to which the counselor responded via interview and observation of program graduates. Some descriptors were simple and clear, such as no insects or bugs present in residence, no frayed appliance wires, and no presence of odors from garbage, laundry, or pets. Others were simply vague and open to wide interpretation, such as an apartment being "reasonably clean."

Many of the problems inherent in New Start's approach to evaluation were embodied in the follow-up evaluation project. For example, the tracking of graduates was viewed as the sole evaluation activity, as opposed to being one component of a broader evaluation plan to assess program outcomes. The narrow scope of the follow-up project and its implementation plan suggested that a broad evaluation policy did not exist for the agency.

Staff Supervision Practices

Even though New Start thought of itself as a place for the novice to gain experience, the agency may have actually provided little in the way of formal training. The frequency and quality of inservice presentations were low, based on reports from informants. During an interview, the senior counselor presented a wish list of topics in which he required instruction. The topics were essential to working in this field: dealing with SSI (Supplemental Security Income) and the Social Security system; a general overview of learning disabilities, including the brain-injured; instructional practices; and psychotherapeutic techniques. There were some kinds of staff supervision at New Start, including clinical supervision and inservice training, however, the frequency of this training as well as its effectiveness was criticized by the senior counselor.

The Role and Effect of a Prominent Leader

Informants who discussed the leadership style of the original director, Darren Mickelson, represented several key perspectives: former employees, including his long-term assistant and evaluator, Dooley; one of his successors, who knew him before and after joining the agency; and a referral agency counselor, who knew him as an external, but involved, professional and who eventually became his subordinate. Each of the informants recognized his leadership skills, especially his ability to generate support for his projects. They described him as dedicated, ambitious, hard-working, strong, and clever. Each informant readily understood how his talents served him and the agency. None of them offered any ideas as to how these same talents may have contributed to the agency's collapse.

During his seven-year tenure the agency grew phenomenally. During that same time, many fundamental problems became apparent, only to remain unresolved under Mickelson's leadership. These included chronic agency-wide problems such as poor staff supervision, low pay for most staff, marginal dwellings for clients, an accelerating rate of staff turnover, and questionable tenant safety. Nevertheless, he successfully maintained the endorsement and support of referral agencies. He left New Start in 1983 to become the director of the State Disabilities Department, the most powerful of those referral agencies.

In the agency's nascent years, Mickelson played a major role in hiring all the staff members at New Start. Data showed that the earliest groups of employees stayed the longest time at the agency, while the time employed for those hired later dropped off considerably. Mickelson's charisma may account, in part, for the large differences in the average number of months employed between those hired in the early years versus those hired in later years. Brief accounts of informants with respect to evaluation and staff supervision policies indicated that, in the later years of his tenure, Mickelson had minimal interest in these administrative areas.

Description of the Sample

The individual profiles of New Start participants differed widely according to age, psychosocial development, functional level, and intact skills. This sample consisted of 15 graduates of the New Start program, six men and nine women, all Caucasian. Table 3 contains data on the sample, ordered by date of entry, with respect to length of time in the program, chronological age, and IQ scores.

TABLE 3

Description of the Sample

Subject	Date In	Date Out	Total Mos.	Age	IQ
S.S.	1980	1982	16	28 yrs.	103
W.B.	1980	1982	17	28 yrs.	unkwn
J.C.	1980	1982	27	35 yrs.	66
D.M.	1981	1983	23	34 yrs.	67
J.L.	1981	1984	36	42 yrs.	unkwn
P.B.	1982	1983	18	27 yrs.	73
A.L.	1982	1983	18	25 yrs.	72
G.M.	1982	1984	21	52 yrs.	82
R.D.	1982	1984	23	21 yrs.	54
A.K.	1982	1984	24	36 yrs.	71
S.G.	1982	1984	24	30 yrs.	68
E.F.	1982	1984	26	24 yrs.	91
I.W.	1982	1984	29	56 yrs.	78
K.L.	1983	1985	16	25 yrs.	unkwn
F.L.	1983	1985	24	42 yrs.	unkwn

The average length of time participants spent in New Start was just under two years, although four remained in the program for one and a half years or less, and four took more than two years to officially complete the program. Ages ranged from 21 to 56 years. The mean age was 33.67 years. Four sample members were older than 40, and four were younger than 25. IQ scores ranged from 103 to 54 on full scale measures. Four of the subjects' IQ scores were not available from their records.

As was typical with all program participants, upon entering the program the subject's skills were evaluated by a team comprised of a New Start staff member, a family member, and a referring counselor. The New Start staff member was responsible for determining the highest level of functioning in all skill areas as specified on the Blue Form by interviewing the other team members and observing the new program participant. The assessment process was expected to be completed within one month.

Basic living skills (i.e., using the bus, cooking and cleaning, shopping alone, doing laundry) seemed to be rated as partially adequate for all subjects (see Table 4). Money management was generally the subjects' greatest weakness, while social deportment seemed to be a common strength. Motivation for all subjects was generally rated high.

TABLE 4

Staff Assessment of Subjects' Skill Levels

	Adequate Skills	Partially Adequate	Inadequate Skills
Basic Skills	0	8	7
Money Management	0	1	14
Housekeeping	5	4	6
Motivation	9	3	3
Social Behavior	6	7	2

Employment histories were poor, especially among the women; three of the men had been competitively employed prior to entering New Start. Housekeeping skills were judged to be adequate, with certain minor deficiencies. The entire sample except for one had associated psychiatric indicators. In fact, four of the subjects, all women, had histories of previous psychiatric episodes. Moreover, every subject had documentation indicating they had either been medicated psychotropically and/or had reported suicidal ideation at some time in the past.

The circumstances that brought the sample members to New Start were probably typical for the majority of participants of independent living skills programs. In the cases of at least 12 subjects, a parent or other family member acting as a parent persuaded the subject to enroll in New Start. In some cases, this persuasion resembled coercion.

It was not unusual for family tragedy to play a pivotal role in the subject's interest in New Start. In at least two cases, the death of a caretaking parent prompted the subject's enrollment. In another case, the financial collapse of a caretaking parent forced a program enrollment. It was apparent in these cases that the parents or the designated caretaking family member were no longer willing to provide primary care for the dependent. One subject came to New Start following an extended period of independent living out of town. He had originally been sent out of town to a pre-arranged job opportunity following his parents' divorce, which had left his mother with two sons and virtually no financial resources.

Only eight of the subjects enrolled in New Start as the result of a friendly mutual agreement with their parents. In one case, the subject's parents relocated to the West Coast so that their daughter could enroll in New Start. One subject elected to leave the program early to marry her boyfriend, who had previously graduated. Fourteen of the subjects officially graduated from the program, participated in the formal graduation ceremony, received certificates, and were considered capable of living independently and, thereby, successful.

Program success was measured by four criteria: the graduate a.) completed an individualized program; b.) demonstrated mastery of living skills as assessed by the Blue Form; c.) had his or her own place to live, alone or with a roommate; and d.) had an active daily schedule that included a work activity, preferably competitive employment. Graduation was a ritualized affair, resembling a traditional school ceremony.

Typically, a resident's schedule was organized by the week. Staff actually distributed single-sheet weekly calendars that the resident and the staff person completed together. The resident was subsequently to continue this practice on his or her own. It was implicit that each resident have enough activities to fill a week. Because few new residents could meet this standard, the program provided a routine from which the individual would hopefully derive a personal schedule. Occupation of the daytime hours was at a premium.

One standard activity was the regular weekly meetings with the staff person, two to three times a week at first, diminishing after several months to once a week. At these meetings the staff person reviewed the resident's calendar, shopping list, weekly meal plan, and so forth. Remedial instruction was provided as needed.

A work schedule had to be included in the week's activities. For the few residents who were competitively employed, their jobs accounted for most of their time. For the majority, work time was arranged and scheduled during regular daytime hours at a volunteer job or at the sheltered workshop. For others, work time was accounted for by participation in a training program. Attendance in classes at the local community college might also account for 1 or 2 days per week. The remaining daytime hours were taken up by doctor's appointments, trips to the market, and other routine, occasional activities.

Evening-hour activities were essentially left to the discretion of the residents unless problems ensued. Typical problems involved sexual activity, the presence of people unknown or disapproved of by staff (e.g., transients or opportunists who might victimize the residents), and excessive use and or abuse of controlled substances. By comparison, social isolation was of less concern because it did not compromise the safety or security of the building or other residents.

Staff did struggle periodically with the question of how much television residents should be allowed to watch, especially if other, more social activities were absent. At times, staff offered evening social groups that presented information of interest to residents, such as contraception, parenting issues, and personal safety. These groups were not intended to act directly as social venues, although this was clearly an unofficial staff agenda item.

Once the resident had been given a final comprehensive evaluation of skills and had met the criteria for graduation as measured by the Blue Form, work began on finding a place to live in the community. Most residents were allowed as much as six months to locate a new residence, but in certain cases graduation was a whirlwind in which the individual was asked to move out even though he might have only his parents' home as a choice.

Using the four program criteria for success, some of the sample members were judged successful (the "Independents"); some just as clearly failed (the "Failures"). Others could not be judged with respect to either success or failure. This last subset, the "Pseudo-Independents," was neither primarily independent nor primarily dependent. Their lifestyles did not easily conform to New Start's expectations, yet they felt and behaved as though they were independent. Their abilities seemed to be limited when compared to the independent group, yet they commanded considerable resources (e.g., family support, their own apartments, financial support), which permitted them to live on their own.

Description of the Research Procedures

Data for this study were collected as part of a more comprehensive investigation into the lives of retarded adults as conducted by the Socio Behavioral Group (SBG) of the UCLA Mental Retardation Research Center. All observations, interviews, and other data were obtained between the years 1979 and 1986. The bulk of observations from 1979 through 1981 were collected as part of the larger SBG research project. The researcher or an associate visited with the selected subjects weekly. From 1981 to 1986 the researcher conducted follow-up interviews and made selected observations with all the subjects at least annually, subject to each subject's willingness to cooperate.

In most cases, participants were cooperative and rapport was established easily. Each participant was presented with a brief description of the research project and advised that participation was a matter of choice and that he or she would be able to withdraw at any point.

Levine (1985) described how, as research subjects, people with mental retardation can be indirect or can show ambivalence in making decisions or choices. The only difficulty with subject rapport encountered in this research involved the willingness of two participants to be interviewed or observed in follow-up, although they had been part of the original sample. Each had originally established rapport with a different investigator and, although they were wary of the new investigator, they were unwilling to be removed as subjects. Rather, they asked the observer to "call back in a few weeks." These invitations were accepted on the subjects' terms, establishing a new, if limited, rapport. Eventually, both subjects provided the observer with lengthy follow-up interviews.

Data were collected in the following formats: a.) participant observations and interviews took place at program sites, participants' living quarters, via telephone conversations, and the homes of participants' family members; b.) staff interviews were conducted at work sites, through telephone conversations, and during informal meetings arranged by the investigator; c.) staff and other peripheral informants agreed to respond to written summaries of observational data verbally and in writing; and d.) agency participant and personnel records were reviewed. One particularly useful data source was provided by the SDD caseworker for seven of the 15 subjects in the sample. He provided written impressions of the key issues he believed were involved in the successful emancipation of these people.

In total, 95 formal observations or interviews were made on the sample. The number of interviews and observations per subject ranged from one to 13. The focus of the interviews and observations varied. Initially, the observer sought to describe the participant's daily routine and the execution of every-day living tasks. Additionally, the observer identified special individual characteristics, including historical and familial information that gave each participant a unique identity. Follow-up interviews focused on the individual's development as a program graduate, especially in terms of his or her own satisfaction with the quality of life.

Some subjects were interviewed and/or observed from six to 18 months after program graduation. The subjects interviewed only once were two couples who were not part of the larger, preliminary investigation and were not known or available to the investigator until quite late. The investigator became aware of these participants after examining agency records and was able to obtain one personal interview and conduct several phone conversations with each couple. Descriptive statistics were compiled from the quantitative data collected on the subjects and agency staff.

Chapter 4

The
_____Independents

Five subjects in this sample clearly established independent and successful lives. They had personal incomes which, for the most part, they managed privately; they lived in their own apartments in the community, unprotected by official agencies; their social lives were anchored in the normal world; they had completely separated from New Start; they maintained supportive relationships with their families but on a carefully limited basis; and they all possessed a fierce desire to be independent, or self-reliant.

Yet, within this group, the qualities of personal happiness, economic and personal stability, employment, satisfaction, friendships, and other aspects of living which all contributed to their perceived success, varied to a great degree.

These five subjects, as with all sample members, are discussed in terms of several categories of information which allow for comparisons to be made between subjects and subject groups. These categories reflect many of the various areas of interest in the field of independent living training as well as provide information in new areas. They include appearance, personal background, current home life, personality, employment status, social life, and parental/family involvement. Possibly, these categories provide a structure for program staff to base a preliminary and follow-up evaluation of successful independent living.

Walter and Stefan

Appearance: Unlike many retarded persons who can easily pass for non-handicapped on the basis of their appearance alone, Stefan, and especially Walter were noticably different. Stefan walked with a stoop and had a prominent scar, wide and long, on his throat from an operation eight years ago. His fingers, in fact all his extremities, were noticably red as though they had been recently soaked in very hot water. Walter had a speech impairment and a hitched walk. When conversing his head dipped and rose in an odd manner. He had a way of staring askance during conversation that was disconcerting at first. Fully animated, Walter's movements suggested a mild cerebral palsy.

Personal Background: The two young men were not natural friends. Prior to enrolling in New Start, Stefan lived a very comfortable life, watched over by his devoted mother in his parents' Beverly Hills home. Walter, on the other hand, lived with his two older brothers in an apartment because his father had suggested they all learn to support themselves. Walter acquired most of his roughneck character during the year he lived with his brothers. In contrast to Stefan's penny loafers and tailored shirts, Walter wore plain t-shirts, smoked Marlboros, drank beer, and used rough language.

Current Home Life: After graduating, the two moved into a two-bedroom apartment in a neighborhood of 10 to 30-unit apartment houses, many of which were home to local university students. They paid $406 a month each for their quarters. During the observation period their building underwent a major facelift, acquiring a security gate and phone system, new paint, and landscaping. Apartment interiors were also refinished, some quite extensively, with the installation of new kitchens and appliances. Stefan and Walter opted not to redo their interior. "We pay $406 each but our apartment is cheaper than the others which go for $925 a month because they have been heavily remodeled. We chose not to remodel in order to keep the rent low. We didn't need to remodel anyway. It's more important to keep the place affordable," they said.

Although they lived in an apartment that was not modern, they did not lack comfort. Together, they commanded an impressive array of electronic equipment. They owned a complete stereo system (turntable, receiver, equalizer, and 4-way speakers), a tape deck, two VCRs (one beta and one VHS), three color TVs with remote control (one in each bedroom plus the living room), and a library of video and audio tapes. The living room wall displayed a gold Beatles album and a collection of Olympic pins. They also owned a telephone answering machine.

A sense of pride and style in their living quarters was evident. The observer was immediately aware that they had done their best to tastefully furnish their apartment. For example, while access to furniture may not have been significantly more advantageous for them than for their fellow graduates, they had made an obvious effort to match the pieces, set the table, and position the cabinets so that everything looked just right.

Personality: Walter and Stefan each possessed an exceptionally enthusiastic spirit. They were members of the community. They went into debt and they pulled themselves out. They had circles of friends with whom they shared activities and interests, all accomplished independent of associations that promote social activities for the developmentally disabled.

Unlike many New Start residents, Stefan was effectively unaware of his status as a handicapped person. Whereas other subjects never seemed to forget, Stefan never recalled. He certainly did not see himself as being held back because of his handicap. When questioned about feeling stigmatized, Stefan responded by saying, "I used to feel that way, like no one would be interested in going out with me. But that is why I decided to go out. Because I didn't want to feel that way anymore. And I don't anymore."

He recalled that the regulars and employees at the bar he frequented once inquired about his funny walk. He simply told them he had some handicaps. Stefan appeared to use the emotional power of stigma as motivation for his adventurous behavior.

Walter also did not recognize himself as handicapped. His concerns were far removed from the limits of being handicapped. "I need a steady girlfriend and a better job, then I'd be real happy. I plan to go back to school next semester. I'd like to get into UCLA and take some business courses to better myself. Maybe get into computers. It's time for me to get a kick-back desk job. Maybe a trade school in computers or anything to get a little more education," Walter said.

Employment: Walter and Stefan were the most successful New Start graduates in this sample. Both graduated from the program early (in 1982), then quickly lost contact with it. Both had remained employed in competitive jobs since graduation although there were times when finances were shaky for each.

Stefan, who had no prior work history before entering New Start, was employed as a switchboard operator in a bank, a job for which he trained through the Department of Rehabilitation. New Start was instrumental in arranging the training. Walter worked as a hospital kitchen helper, also a job held since leaving New Start.

Social Life: Throughout the observations, Walter and Stefan demonstrated characteristic enthusiasm in their pursuit of a social life. Their contact with other New Start participants was most frequent when they first graduated. They regularly hosted dinner parties for several guests displaying their imagination and attention to detail.

Stefan disclosed that he loved to cook things like cheese cake and fancy chicken dishes. In preparation of such a meal, he carefully selected an extensive array of fresh produce (raspberries, strawberries, pineapple, cantaloupe, oranges, and apples) for a fruit salad which he planned to make for friends that evening. He also carefully selected a varied group of fresh vegetables (mushrooms, spinach, celery, and avocados) for the salad.

Stefan and Walter were very sociable and both were successful in obtaining friends. Their skills in creating comfort or feeling comfortable in a social environment set Walter and Stefan apart from most of the other subjects. Their dinner parties allowed them to polish their hosting and cooking skills.

As they separated from the program, their satisfaction with hosting these dinners waned, especially in Stefan's case. They each began to see less of their New Start friends and, instead, sought new ways to be a part of the community. Even their own friendship took a back seat to independent quests for new friends. Stefan found new friendship opportunites in his Westwood bank job.

At the beginning of the observations, Stefan made a clear statement about his personal goals; to break all ties with New Start, meet new people, and be completely independent. A year later he explained what motivated him and described some of the results. "I just got tired of sitting in front of the

TV every night. I began going upstairs from work to the bar. I met a couple of girls and became friends with everyone. Now it's my hangout. I've been to the movies with a couple of the waitresses. There's no romance but I'm working on it," Stefan said.

As Stefan widened his circle of friends, Walter felt abandoned, but not stranded without resources. He seemed to be envious of Stefan's new friends from work. He expressed his envy as a serious concern for Stefan's eagerness to be accepted. According to Walter, Stefan was hanging out with a fast crowd, spending a great deal of money he didn't have, and going out every night after work.

The friendship survived the strain of competing pursuits with some interesting results. Walter got involved with a local football booster club, eventually becoming their "mascot," attending numerous games for free. Stefan, meanwhile, incurred a large debt having used his credit cards to pick up nightly drinking tabs with his new bank friends. Stefan's indebtedness and subsequent relief from debt provided valuable learning experiences which contributed to his maturity, sense of responsibility, and independence. Rapidly going into credit-card debt provided Stefan with a meaningful experience in coping with a problem encountered in everyday life. As suggested by Levine (1985), the ability of mentally retarded persons to solve their own problems demonstrates competence and helps maintain self-esteem.

Stefan carefully shielded his parents from his crisis. Instead, he spoke to his friend, a loan officer at the bank, who advised him to secure a bank loan at an employee's loan rate and eliminate two credit cards. He did this incurring payments of $115 a month at 14 percent interest instead of 20 percent. With a mixture of remorse and relief he commented, "I'll have them paid off in three years."

To Walter's credit, he permitted Stefan to solve his own problems, instead of involving an authority figure. Stefan subsequently sought other haunts where he felt less pressured to behave as though he had unlimited funds.

Walter had several circles of friends; from his apartment building, his workplace, and the Booster Club. His friendships, like Stefan's, were not based on sharing handicaps but, rather, were founded in recreation and enjoyment. Walter was a regular bowler, meeting friends informally on certain nights at a local bowling alley. Additionally, he had purchased a 10-speed bike and found people with whom he could ride by the beach on weekends. Since undertaking bike riding he had become more health conscious cutting his smoking down to four cigarettes a day.

While Walter and Stefan were dependent on each other for both companionship and security, they had developed separate and independent lifestyles. The importance of their friendship was evident to each of them as well as to their families. In 1984, when Walter experienced financial difficulties, it appeared that he might be forced to move to a less expensive apartment. The parents of both young men wanted them to stay together. They believed that the partnership of Walter and Stefan was a crucial factor, not only in their initial survival, but also in their continued success.

Parental/Family Involvement: For both Walter and Stefan, the involvement of their parents was helpful, although each involvement was uniquely different. Walter had a supportive relationship with his father. From Walter's point of view, it improved whenever he was not receiving financial support from his father.

For example, during the financial crisis Walter was forced to ask for monetary help for about ten months. His work hours had been cut back severely and he could not raise his entire rent. Walter was given an extra $150 to $200 monthly by his father in order to stay in the apartment. The money was not a gift but was drawn from Walter's trust account. There were two problems with the arrangement, which Walter pointed out: once this money ran out, he expected no further support; and, second, Walter did not know how much money was in the account so he could not estimate how long he could depend on it. Walter felt the information was being withheld by his father, a circumstance which he disliked. He lost his ability to plan for his future as well as to provide for his present lifestyle.

Six months passed before Walter was able to generate more income by finding a part-time job in a warehouse. Four months later, the hospital returned him to a full-time schedule. Walter decided to keep the part-time job as he had become used to the additional income. With two incomes, Walter was netting about $950/month. However, he complained of working too hard to enjoy any rewards. Additionally, he informed the observer that he had no intention of declaring his extra income. He explained that his uncle did his annual taxes, as though his uncle had made the initial suggestion. He declared imploringly, "Uncle Sam is killing me with taxes!"

Walter thought having to return back home would be "a lousy and unhappy experience." It would crush a person's spirit to return home once they had lived on their own. Running out of money on a regular basis made it easy to resume a dependent lifestyle. Without cash, he reflected, one had to leave his own apartment, ask for charity, and "would probably get too lazy to cook." There were no shortcuts to independence. "Either you make it straight or you don't make it at all. Scamming and hustling like Helena (a failed participant) did to stay out on your own is as bad as moving home. There is a drop-off in skills. (She) was very dirty and messy like she had never learned a thing in New Start."

Summary: Both young men grudgingly recognized that New Start deserved some credit for their happy, successful lives. Walter was in New Start 16 months and claimed he had more skills than they could teach him when he arrived. "I did learn how to cook and take buses. I want to get a car again. I'm going to talk to my Dad next week about taking driving lessons."

Upon entering New Start, Walter's general skills were judged adequate. Money management was rated as his greatest area of deficiency. For Walter, being matched with Stefan was probably his greatest program benefit.

Stefan wanted work training so New Start placed him in a sheltered workshop which, in retrospect, was ludicrous. He complained to the staff that he was capable of more and was subsequently placed in the state-funded work-training program which prepared him to work as a switchboard operator (a line of work which, unfortunately, is fast becoming obsolete). Still, it can be argued that the chief benefit Walter and Stefan received from New Start was the chance to become roommates and friends and develop their social skills to a superior level of sophistication.

The Daltons

Appearance: Like Walter and Stefan, the Daltons also looked different, however, this was more a function of their grooming rather than any obvious physical deficit. Both were in their early 20s. Randy was tall and noticeably gaunt with long, thick, oily hair, and thick glasses. Leigh was short, chubby, and also wore glasses. She had thick, kinky black hair, and a smiling, mischievous face full of large freckles. Her personal hygiene was even poorer than Randy's. Her fingernails were profoundly dirty while his were chewed to the tips.

Leigh was quite gregarious, often answering before, if not for, her husband. Randy's and Leigh's IQ scores were well below normal (his was lowest in the sample), yet they demonstrated a mixture of wisdom, immaturity, childish exuberance, and fundamental street-sense. These qualities were discovered only after getting past their appearances which were off-putting.

Personal Background: The Daltons met through the New Start program. It seems unlikely that they could have done as well without each other. Randy and Leigh Dalton married while still enrolled in New Start. Even though they were strongly lobbied to wait until after their graduation, they steadfastly refused to bend to the program's will. When interviewed, they had been married two years. The story of how they prevailed by stubbornly insisting on doing things their way showcased their combined sense of personal power and self-confidence. Leigh said, "It was rocky getting married because we had to get stuck twice for blood tests and the license cost $30 which isn't cheap! New Start wanted us to wait until after we graduated but we didn't want to, so we threatened to elope! We were going to Vegas! We ended up getting married with everyone's agreement anyway. We got married in a church with our family and friends. The New Start staff gave us that poster (on the wall)."

Current Home Life: Together, the Daltons were quite resourceful. They lived together before getting married, and found their apartment by themselves (which was a point of personal pride). The one-bedroom, one-bath apartment was located in a decent neighborhood in Los Angeles' San Fernando Valley.

The building was a large, multiple-unit dwelling. Their well-furnished apartment held an abundance of electronic equipment and belongings including a late-model color TV, a tape deck, additional stereo equipment such as speakers and a turntable, numerous records, many cassette tapes, and a collection of sports hats. The equally cluttered bedroom held three large and very handsome dressers, a queen-size mattress, another late model color TV, luggage, briefcases, and clothes.

Clothes, magazines, and papers were generally strewn about. His and hers bicycles (wedding gifts from her family) were stored on the patio, secured by a heavy, expensive-looking lock. While the place appeared stuffed, it was somehow in order. The apartment was so small it could only be furnished in one basic configuration and still allow for simple movement, which they had accomplished.

Their rent was $400 monthly which they had tried to supplement via a federal housing assistance program, commonly referred to as section 8. Leigh stated that they had been turned down for section 8 once because Randy made too much money. She also informed the observer that they were appealing the denial. The fact that they felt entitled to challenge the decision of the housing agency, and understood their stake in this effort, was an example of their worldliness and confidence. When the observer asked how much money Randy made, Leigh discretely responded, "I don't want to say. It is better to keep that personal and private." It was quite likely that their parents assisted as guides in the interactions with the housing agency.

Leigh realized that joining New Start and marrying Randy made it possible for her to move out of her parents' home, something she had wanted very much. She also credited New Start with helping Randy learn how to shop for new clothes, and groceries, budget money, and use a bank. Leigh did not concur with New Start's initial assessment of her own skills; i.e. inadequate in all the major skill areas. She was unwilling to acknowledge that New Start had taught her any basic skills such as cooking, budgeting, or housekeeping. Nevertheless, both agreed that New Start improved their ability to work as a coordinated team in the kitchen. When they prepared a pot roast in a crockpot, for example, they divided the job into tasks which could be shared. Randy's job was to prepare and supervise the crockpot. In a boastful manner, he pointed out that he put in the right amount of water with the meat. Leigh was responsible for adding vegetables, salt, pepper, and, later on, garlic. The previous night they had made burritos. Once a week they shopped together for groceries.

Personality: Leigh felt that New Start helped improve control of her temper. She claimed that she lost her temper very easily and would often throw tantrums which she described as horrible. "I'm half Armenian and that's the bad side you don't want to get too upset!"

As a couple, Leigh and Randy provided a fascinating example of "false incompetence;" that is, they were simply not as inept as one might assume. They repeatedly dispelled the observer's biases. Although very young, they seemed unexpectedly worldwise, especially about their rights and goals. They were open yet discreet whether discussing sexual practices, banking and bill-paying procedures, income or joyful feelings of independence.

Employment: Randy had been working at the Veteran's Administration as a dishwasher for three or four years, even before New Start. Leigh felt New Start had not helped her secure employment, and she remained unemployed, "(Prior to the program) I had a few jobs and they all flopped." Agency notes showed that Leigh had been counseled that her quick temper was a liability.

She had trained at the West Valley Occupational Center but had never worked at anything other than volunteer positions. She almost didn't graduate from New Start when the program director refused to bend the rules and authorize her graduation without a job. She enrolled at a sheltered workshop since New Start accepted that as a minimum graduation criterion. Even though she felt she did not belong with the people at the sheltered workshop, whom she disdained, she played along until she graduated, after which she promptly quit. Leigh offered a harsh comment on the legitimacy of sheltered workshops as jobs. "Those aren't real jobs anyway." Between SSI payments and his earnings (approximately $6/hour), they netted about $1800 a month.

Social Life: The Daltons appeared to be the most well-to-do couple in the sample. A monetary windfall (a large backpayment of SSI money cited below) had significantly contributed to their level of material comfort as well as their sense of independence. Randy's steady employment was enough to sustain their quality of life. They had plenty of cash to spend as their collection of consumer goods demonstrated.

As Leigh saw it, their main regret was the absence of an active social life. Their best friends were another successful New Start couple (the Larsens, to be discussed with the Pseudo-Independents), but Leigh strongly desired more exciting companions.

Leigh believed she needed to occupy her free time while Randy was working. She missed him during the day and would have liked to increase their income even though she regarded it as comfortable. The two depended on each other for friendship and entertainment. Their unexpected willingness to talk about awkward subjects such as parenting and sex made it clear how committed they were to depending on each other for their futures.

"We have decided against children," Leigh declared for the couple. "They are too costly. Randy has decided to have a vasectomy, probably after the holidays. Right now we practice birth control by not having sex! No, we have oral sex only. No intercourse. New Start taught us about oral sex in the sex education course. We saw slides and talked about it. It was embarrassing!"

In their minds, they were finished with New Start. Leigh gleefully shouted her feelings about their independence. "We kids are free! We do whatever we want!" They were living comfortably and claimed to enjoy their lives. At the time, their short-term goal was a week's vacation in Hawaii. They planned to cut expenses by staying with Randy's sister, who was living there. Leigh added that Randy could use some of his vacation time. Her eyes widened as she marveled that Randy could get paid to go on a vacation to Hawaii.

Parental/Family Involvement: The Daltons received help from their parents at critical points in life. As with Stefan and Walter, when the Daltons needed help, it was provided by parents in the form of monetary loans and gifts. Leigh told how a new Social Security caseworker had mistakenly cut off their SSI for four months. The worker's error forced them to borrow money from her parents, which they would have rather avoided. Once their benefits were reinstated, they received a large check in backpay which they used, in part, to reimburse Leigh's parents. They were proud to pay her parents back. Leigh made sure their files were transferred to another caseworker.

Leigh did not discuss her relationship with her parents in great detail, but said enough to reveal ambivalent feelings. She was glad to be free of them, yet she trusted their counsel and financial protection. For example, Randy and Leigh received several gifts of money for their wedding. Her parents suggested she allow her brother to hold the funds in an account in his name, thereby shielding the money from SSI. They agreed to the arrangement.

Summary: The Daltons' discrete yet candid responses consistently uncovered prejudices held by the observer. For example, the observer had presumed that if independence was hard to achieve for a single person, it would be next to impossible for a couple. In addition, the Daltons' low IQ scores and poor skills upon entry to New Start had suggested to the observer that the couple would struggle to keep afloat. Instead, the observer found a strong partnership, united in the fight to choose their own destiny, and enjoy married life on their own terms. Such terms included an implicit demand that important information not be withheld from them simply because it was presumed they were incapable of understanding.

The observer's tendency to discount the Daltons' potential for success was quickly replaced by an urge to render them heroic. It was easy to imagine them as the ideal retarded couple; independently forging their united path in life, disarming skeptics with their frankness, discretion, and common sense. Enshrining the Daltons, however, was as unfair as prejudging them. Their happiness and success were built on the strength of their own friendship and love. Randy valued Leigh's gregariousness and she thrived on his enthusiastic support for her. They managed to create a life they believed was filled with love, excitement, and comfort.

Janice

Appearance: In the parlance of her own SDD worker, Janice was a "funny looking kid." The worker explained that this meant one could make a judgment about normalcy on appearance alone.

Personal Background: Janice was a single woman in her mid-30s. She was the second oldest of four; the others being normal and successful. Her parents lived in Beverly Hills, enjoyed great personal success, and both held advanced degrees. Her father was a world-reknowned endocrinologist who lectured at universities across Europe and the Americas. Janice was raised and cared for by her mother who, according to Janice and others, was her closest friend and principal ally. Janice graduated from Beverly Hills High School.

Current Home Life: Janice graduated from New Start in 1981, after 27 months in the program, with full program endorsement and a bank job in walking distance from her home. According to her Blue Form, she had mastered laundry, grocery shopping, and banking. Observations in the four months immediately following her graduation revealed she still had problems with cooking and housekeeping. It could not be determined if she had actually mastered banking since she stated that her mother handled all those tasks for her.

Her program apartment was a hodgepodge of articles, with very little concern for matching furniture or colors, or for maintaining regular upkeep. Many of her things were falling apart or badly ripped. She blamed her roommate's cat for the tattered couch and chairs.

The observer was surprised the living room was so unkempt and messy since the New Start counselors were supposed to monitor cleanliness. The kitchen was another clutter of odd pots and pans and empty cupboards. The sink was full of dirty dishes. The burner wells and trivets on the stove were very greasy. The bathroom was more of the same. There was one grundgy handtowel on the rack and the tub was moldy and dirty. The mirror had several weeks of film on it.

Janice explained to the observer that her roommate rarely cleaned. Janice tended to fix blame elsewhere. After four months of observations during which the state of her apartment remained unchanged, it was apparent that Janice also did little cleaning.

One task which she accomplished with little complaint or difficulty was laundry. She performed laundry tasks with no problems and uncharacteristic confidence. This contrasted with her more typical behavior; experiencing so much stress in a routine task that she became incapable of accomplishing it without help. As an example, a shopping trip for which she appeared anxious, deteriorated rapidly:

> Janice was the picture of disorganization in her preparation to go shopping. She attributed this to having just arrived home from work; having had a rough day sorting checks (at her bank job); and having misplaced her shopping list from the night before. She struggled with the decision to cancel shopping, to make a new list, or to go without a list. She decided to take a quick look around the kitchen, make a quick list, and go ahead with the trip. She had a wallet full of money from cashing her paycheck that day and had to decide how much to take with her. As with many subjects, she decided on the amount of money to take based on how much would be needed to cover any unforeseen costs. In the market she went about the shopping very slowly, stopping to deliberate on every item. She spoke out loud in the market, attracting

attention. She questioned whether the food was good for her, too expensive, too large a quantity, etc. She ended up abandoning her list almost immediately. She said she always bought the same things anyway. In the checkout line, she paid the cashier very slowly reminding the observer that she must save money to move out (after graduating New Start) and would need 'every penny I have'. (excerpt from field notes)

Exactly what stressed Janice so greatly about taking a trip to buy food was unclear, but her tendency to deteriorate under pressure was a daily event, occuring under numerous conditions (from shopping to working), reported by numerous sources (herself, her SDD worker, the observer, and her bank supervisor).

Personality: Janice's SDD worker wrote that Janice's personality was just as much a handicap as her diagnosis of mild mental retardation. The worker contended that Janice had a history of isolation among her peers, failing to generate friendships in all social settings, including high school and New Start. Her SDD worker made the following comments:

> Her paranoid and rigid personality did not allow for much success at friendship. . .She is used to being unaccepted but will not allow her rigid defense system down for one moment. She refuses and is, perhaps, incapable of exploring the reasons for her consistent failures (in friendships) and rejections.

The worker described her participation in New Start as attentive and somewhat successful. Yet, the worker believed that the quality of Janice's life was compromised by her significant personality problems:

> Janice was almost autistic-like in the way she dealt with other New Start participants. . .like a robot asking the expected appropriate questions. . .her emotionless style of interacting. . .(she) would become extremely defensive at any suggestion that she was not performing as expected. . .(she was) a difficult one for the staff. . .her rigidity and defensiveness took precedence whenever a new task or positive criticism was presented.

Janice was described by her SDD worker as a powerful victim who sought being rescued by others whether it was in relieving her indecision about meal preparation, or in getting her New Start counselor to request that her bank supervisor criticize her less frequently. "As the victim, Janice does not sit and wait. She does not view herself as helpless. Rather, she compulsively asks for help. . . ."

To her SDD worker, Janice's ritualistic style of asking for help seemed to be an integral part of her personality. By delaying decision making when anxious, Janice successfully compelled others to assist her. By passively enlisting the help of others she simultaneously found relief from her performance anxiety. Her successful and constant attempts to elicit the help of others by delaying decision making was documented in nearly every observation of Janice.

The observer, for example, was caught up in the effect during a scheduled observation of her cooking skills. She had made no preparation for a meal that was to be observed and she was upset. She had many work-related stories about how she worked fast enough here but not fast enough there. She did not have enough food for a meal and complained that she had too much to do to get ready for the meal. Visibly agitated, she puzzled over three possible decisions: canceling the meal; shopping for food; or putting something together from odds and ends in her cupboard and refrigerator. She voiced concern that her performance was embarrassing.

Finally the observer intervened as she grew more agitated and directionless. With his coaxing she chose to prepare a meal from her cupboard; spaghetti, string beans, corn, and Pepsi. She still could not produce a successful meal. She stumbled through the task of assembling a meal from leftovers. For salad, she threw a can of tuna into a bowl of beans and corn. She tossed the spaghetti into a pot of cold water. After voicing continual distress and anxiety, she suggested that she simply buy them hamburgers.

Janice found a remedy for her anxiety by regularly citing claims of independence which functioned like chants of affirmation. These affirmations frequently occurred after a crisis, and may have helped reduce her level of stress. Common affirmations included statements related to building herself up for living on her own, securing work, and getting promotions.

Social Life: Her most current report of social activities centered around two social groups; one organized by parents' of retarded adults, and one by her parents' temple. When pressed to describe her favorite leisure activities, the more familiar picture of isolation, blended with her characteristic optimism, emerged. Janice said:

> I like to go to movies or browse and go shopping. I usually go alone when I do those things. I have had a driver's license for a couple of years but have no plans to get a car. It is just too expensive, at least that is what my parents say. They tend to play down the idea of me getting a car. It is too expensive. . .I am very close with my parents. I also think I am more independent than ever. . .I have no romantic involvements at the moment and no plans either for the time being.

Employment: Despite her personality and social deficits, Janice was considered to be successful for two reasons. She lived on her own in a very attractive section of the city, and she was usually employed in a competitive job. Even though she frequently lost jobs, she was adroit at finding new work on short notice.

At the time of the last observation, Janice was still working, although no longer at the bank. She was a busgirl at a lunchstop in Santa Monica. She rode the bus to work every day. She was vague when describing her new position, making it sound like a managerial position. She claimed she was responsible for opening up the place and getting the whole operation ready for the day's business. Further inquiry established that she prepared the dining room by setting tables, arranging chairs, and placing salt and pepper shakers on the tables before the customers arrived.

She discussed her income freely, with the familiar blend of affirmation and exaggeration:

> I learned a lot. You know, living independently. I was recently promoted at my job. I got the job through New Start. I work at the (lunch stop) in the new building at (a certain corner). I get $291.92 every two weeks. I am expecting a raise but it might not be for a couple of weeks. I also get Social Security—$453 a month.

Parental/Family Involvement: Of particular importance was the support Janice's parents provided at critical points in her life. They were instrumental in helping Janice obtain the cornerstone of her independent lifestyle—a condominium located near a thriving commercial and entertainment district. Once Janice and her roommate had officially graduated from New Start they found themselves in the awkward position of waiting to exit the program's apartment for one they had yet to find. Several months passed without results. During this transitional period Janice's roommate was murdered. The crime was especially frightening to Janice and her parents because the roommate was killed in the apartment (Janice was not home). Janice's parents responded swiftly and conclusively. They purchased a one-bedroom, one-bath security condominium in a wealthy section of town.

Janice also had received a windfall payment from SSI; about $10,000 in retroactive payments. She reported that the lump payment followed a dispute settled in her favor over prior termination of benefits.

Her SDD worker stated that Janice had underreported her earnings and had been issued the check under false pretenses. Janice furnished her new condo with some of the money and kept the rest in the bank. SSI countersued her for the money. Janice insisted that she had done nothing wrong and that the SSI system was at fault. Her worker stated Janice's argument was nothing more than protest and denial and suspected that her parents had played a major role in the entire affair.

Janice was especially dependent on her parents where money was concerned. Her mother handled all the banking even though Janice once worked in a bank. The following quote from Janice revealed how her parents had arranged for her to pay very little rent while appearing to pay almost $1,000 as well as possibly to conceal the fact that her own parents owned her apartment:

> My paycheck goes to my Mom. I see her every week. She also deposits my Social Security check in my checking account. They know me at my bank and help me out a lot. Mainly my parents do my banking. My rent is $250 a month for a one-bedroom and one-bath apartment. My parents are friends with the landlords. Once a month I also sign a check for my dad for $700 to the landlords. Then I sign mine for $250. They get both. I don't bounce checks anymore.

Summary: Janice's life was, like herself, an odd mix of contradictions which seemed to result in a parade of struggles. In her interactions with others she frequently set herself up as a victim, yet she acted powerfully in many of these relationships.

Her achievements in establishing friendships, keeping jobs, and directing her own life were marginal, at best. With her mother's assistance she continued to plunge ahead in life, determined to be on her own, especially in her own mind. Her strongest claim to independence was the very belief that she was independent and self-reliant.

SECTION SUMMARY:
THE INDEPENDENTS

Independence for this group was viewed as hierarchical, with Stefan and Walter providing the strongest examples, and Janice the weakest. The lifestyles of all five individuals had qualities which fundamentally distinguished them from the other sample members, as well as each other.

All rapidly separated from the New Start program following graduation. They all depended on their parents for financial help, even though this seemed to be limited to crisis situations. For example, Walter needed help for several months when his work hours were cut back. Janice's parents purchased her condo after her roommate was murdered. The Daltons allowed their parents to suggest a way to shield their income from SSI, but otherwise, preferred to control their own funds. While Stefan created his own credit card debt, he also solved it on his own.

Four of the five had strong work histories and, during the observation period, held competitive jobs. Leigh was the sole exception, benefiting from husband Randy's well-paying, secure federal job. On the other hand, she handled all their money.

All five entered New Start unable to balance their checkbooks and all five graduated that way. The skills which this group acquired during their tenure at New Start seemed to have been mixed, if not marginal. They possessed substantial living skills when they entered the program, so their level of traditional living skills did not seem to be an element which distinguished them, either from the others or among themselves.

The role of parents or other significant helpers is a form of dependence first identified by Edgerton (1967). The five subjects seemed to differ among each other most clearly on this matter. Walter and Stefan, and Randy and Leigh preferred to keep their parents at a safe distance, using them peripherally, maintaining a strong boundary which effectively limited intrusion. Stefan and Walter were more sure about the importance of this boundary than were Randy and Leigh, although both "couples" allowed much less parental contact and management than Janice. She (like the next ten subjects remaining to be discussed) allowed her parents to take a significantly greater role in her life. Most telling was her mother's control of her money. In allowing her mother to deposit her checks, Janice gave up her privacy and, subsequently, basic control of her funds.

By comparison, Walter accepted monthly payments through his father, from his own savings, in order to supplement his income during a money crisis. Like Janice, he had only nominal control, not even knowing how much he had in that account. Like Walter, Janice wrote her own checks and paid her own bills, but she gave up her privilege to control her funds permanently and privately as long as her mother received her statements. This arrangement supposedly existed because Janice could not adequately handle the check register. The degree to which her mother intruded into Janice's life distinguished her from the others in her subgroup, positioning her closer to the less independent subjects.

Finally, Janice's personality was the most disturbing of the group. She was reclusive, somewhat paranoid, and doggedly ignorant of her own role in her job troubles. Stefan and Walter were decidedly the opposite. They were uniformly enthusiastic about life, socially charming, and typically open-minded about their difficulties in life.

Randy and, especially, Leigh were more like Stefan and Walter than like Janice in psychological adjustment. Leigh's temper and obvious insecurity about her ability to hold a job made her the second most disturbing personality among the group. However, Randy's benign and cooperative presence seemed to stabilize her anger and depression.

This balance of personal liabilities and assets provided Randy and Leigh with an advantage over Janice, whose best friend was her mother. Janice's mother did not provide a balance to her life, instead assuming major responsibilities for her daughter's life as a partial solution to Janice's problems.

The phenomenon of personality characteristics acting as obstacles in securing independence became more of an issue for each successive subject within this group. Correspondingly, the inability of the New Start program to address these issues became more apparent.

Chapter 5

The Pseudo-
_____Independents

Seven New Start graduates in the sample considered themselves to be independent, even though there was much dependence evident in their lifestyles. These graduates lived in their own apartments and carried out their daily living chores of laundry, cooking, shopping, and transportation without the assistance or guidance of others.

There were two couples within this group; one platonic and one romantic. However, only one subject held a competitive job, although four others regularly maintained work-like routines at volunteer jobs. All were involved with their families to a greater extent than the Independent group.

The Pseudo-Independent subjects struggled to balance dependence and independence in their lives. Unlike the Independent subjects, their struggle was rarely resolved or mediated without compromises made between themselves and their parents (or parental figures). In each case, these compromises seemed to favor dependence more than independence. Additionally, it became evident that psychological factors weighed more heavily in the explanation of each Pseudo-Independent subject's state of affairs.

The Larsens

Appearance: Francis was 41 years old, and approximately 5'1" in height. His body was round, with a squat torso perched above bandy legs, and a remarkably oblong head. He wore glasses. He was married to Kristy, who was 24 years old, about three inches taller than Francis, equally plump, with noticably bad skin on her round, wide-eyed face. She wore thick glasses beneath her messy, short black hair. Kristy and Francis looked retarded.

Personal Background: Francis and Kristy met in the New Start program. Francis entered the program four months earlier than Kristy, graduating after 24 months while Kristy dropped out four months prior to her scheduled graduation.

Francis had a long-standing relationship with his cousin Roy who had acted as Francis' caretaker before Francis was placed in New Start. According to Francis, Roy dissented on the New Start decision, preferring that Francis remain in a board and care facility. It was Francis' sister who placed him in New Start. While Francis also resisted the idea, he hated the board and care home even more.

Kristy said she had learned a little about cooking from her mother prior to entering New Start, but knew little else about living on her own. She credited New Start with teaching her how to cook, use a bank, budget, and become more independent. Kristy did not graduate from New Start, electing to get married instead. New Start wanted her to graduate before marrying, and advised her that she could not continue in the program if she didn't comply. This ultimatum, along with her anger that her counselors had been switched too often, comprised her primary complaints about the program.

Current Home Life: The Larsens lived together in a large apartment complex (approximately 100 units) across from a public park which was more of a haven for the homeless than a resource for the neighborhood. Their one-bedroom apartment on the third floor had a kitchen that flowed into an open dining area which in turn emptied into a living area. Their bedroom was on the other side of the kitchen wall. They weren't as skilled in decorating as some other subjects, but they did keep a neat household.

The living and dining areas were somewhat cluttered with an impressive collection of electronic equipment, including a TV, VCR, cassette tape player, TV cable-channel selector, another tape to tape player, numerous records and tapes, and many loose and framed personal photographs displayed on shelves between the machines. Most of the equipment sat amidst a menagerie of stuffed animals on a very large and crowded living room shelf unit. Their walls were decorated with several paintings including one of Elvis Presley on black velvet.

A large leaded-glass coffee table anchored the living room. The dining room table, like the coffee table, was too big for the dining area adjoining the kitchen. As a result, walking into the kitchen required careful maneuvering. The kitchen showed more dirt than the living and dining area. The Larsens had roaches which they said were to be exterminated the following month. They claimed they owned all their appliances including the stove, refrigerator, toaster, and electric can opener. In their bedroom was a late model 25-inch color TV.

Personality: Francis behaved nervously. He was easily excited, and seemed prone to impulsive behavior. Kristy's behavior was similar but more flamboyant. For example, with obvious excitement, she spontaneously challenged the observer to an arm wrestling match. This was spontaneous and completely unrelated to any conversation or activity.

Francis seemed like someone who could be easily intimidated, by both his wife and cousin. Both acknowledged that they were fundamentally dependent on cousin Roy, a relationship which they valued and resented. Kristy disliked having to go to Roy for their money, but recognized the importance of his assistance in times of crisis.

Employment: Francis worked at Roy's McDonalds as a fry cook. The restaurant was close to his home. Roy had arranged for Francis to work there 21 hours a week, although Francis actually was paid in cash as undeclared wages for the other 19 hours. The deception was for the benefit of SSI, so that their benefits would not be jeopardized.

The Larsen's monthly income approximated $1,300, including Francis' $177 from McDonalds every two weeks; another $200 monthly in undeclared cash wages from McDonalds; and $400 a month each from SSI.

Social Life: The Larsens dated for nine months, lived together for one year, then married in June 1985. Their major goal in life, according to them, was to fight boredom. Francis worked during the day while Kristy stayed home with nothing to do. In the evenings they watched TV till they got bored, then worked on several jigsaw puzzles which remained partially assembled in the living and dining rooms. Francis claimed he used to drink quite heavily in the past, and regarded alcohol abuse as a danger of boredom.

Parental/Family Involvement: Cousin Roy was responsible for Francis' employment and was deeply involved in the couple's financial management. In the past year he had helped Francis out of a serious dispute with SSI. According to Francis, he had sued for benefits which had been discontinued for the two previous years. He won a judgment resulting in retroactive payments of nearly $10,000. However, the judgment stipulated that he have a legal guardian. With Roy acting as guardian, the Larsens (like the Daltons) used the money to purchase their freedom. Some of the money was used to get married and honeymoon in Hawaii.

Once they returned, they quickly incurred a debt crisis which they attributed to a puzzling, yet believable, directive from their SSI worker which compelled them to spend the cash as quickly as possible or face being disqualified for SSI benefits once again. In order to spend the remaining $6,000 they purchased furniture and stereo equipment, much of it on credit or COD. Francis wrote checks when the bills arrived until he had overdrawn the account funded by his cousin by $5,000.

Francis never used a checkbook prior to entering New Start nor did he and Kristy master checking accounts before leaving the program. Cousin Roy took over Francis' account when it became clear that Francis had attempted to conceal the crisis from Roy. A system was established by Roy for the Larsens to draw capital from Roy's secretary every two weeks. Kristy said, "It's just like Project New Start. We still aren't independent."

In Francis' and Kristy's minds, cousin Roy exerted too much control over their lives. They felt like his prisoners, even though by their own account, he was genuinely committed to their welfare. They had complete health insurance through Roy's business which paid for the medical expenses not covered by MediCal, all coordinated by Roy's secretary.

This kindness saved Francis and Kristy much trouble as well as expense, yet it only made Kristy want her freedom even more. "We want to be completely on our own. Roy gets in the way by taking care of Francis too much. And he also yells at Francis a lot." Francis added, "I try to stay out of Roy's way."

Summary: Cousin Roy was the primary figure in the Larsens' lives. Both the couple and the benefactor viewed the relationship as unwanted, but unavoidable. The Larsens' lives centered around their dependence on him. Roy, it seemed, was searching for the least troublesome arrangement to keep the Larsens safe, secure, and happy. The Larsens were cooperative, but felt like Roy's vassals. No one seemed to possess the confidence that Francis and Kristy could really achieve independence.

Ida and Grace

Appearance: Grace was a short, round woman who looked her age of 52 years. Ida also looked her age, 56, and had flaming red hair. Grace wore her light brown and gray hair in a simple, straight cut brushed to the side. Her round face featured sloping eyes, drooping lids, and a mouth that remained partly opened. Ida had a wide, open face with large expressive eyes. Her manner was very congenial bordering on coquettish. Ida's apartment bedroom was "decorated like a young teenage girl's with pink covers and stuffed animals all over the bed. It was a detailed look that clearly suggested adolescence." Ida often wore leather braces on her wrists as her doctor ordered (an independent investigator reported that this was a fabrication). Both women dressed casually in blouses and jeans or pants, paying little attention to style.

Personal Background: Ida had lived with her parents until her father died of old age. After her father's death, her mother Verna decided she could no longer care for Ida and made arrangements to enroll her in New Start. Ida was 56 years old and had been enrolled in the New Start program for four months when observations began. Her enthusiasm for the program was like that of a child going away to summer camp for the first time. In fact, she was childlike in many ways and New Start was her first experience away from home.

Grace had also lived with her parents all her life until they died of natural causes, leaving her alone in the house for several months until she injured herself in a fall. Following this incident, Grace agreed with her sister Rachel to enroll in New Start.

It took Ida 29 months to get through New Start, the longest of all participants in the sample. Although Grace joined the program eight months after Ida, they graduated together. Until Grace's arrival, the New Start staff had been unable to place Ida with a roommate who could tolerate her. It was felt by program staff that Ida's program success hinged on this single issue; finding someone who could live with her. The arrangement proved equally beneficial for Grace.

Current Home Life: Ida and Grace continued to live together after graduating from New Start. They located an apartment that enabled them to walk to the grocery store, the bus, or the corner liquor store. Everything they needed was within reach. Their bus line took them directly to most of their destinations, requiring no transfers.

Ida was quite happy. She was pleased with her weekly activities, apartment, and roommate. She considered herself to be successfully independent. She still couldn't balance her checkbook, but happily pointed out that her life was full. She had her doctors, psychotherapist, and job counselor.

Unfortunately, Grace was at her limit with Ida. After five years with her, the soft-spoken Grace was threatening to terminate the partnership. Her complaints were few but serious. Grace was tired of doing all the cleaning in the apartment. She had decided to neither badger Ida to clean up more often, nor clean up in front of her. In fact, because Ida refused to clean the tub or shower after using it, Grace and Ida had stopped bathing or showering entirely.

Finally, Grace complained that Ida had become physically aggressive with her. This mainly occurred in the mornings as Ida had grown increasingly cross with Grace who was slower to rise. Ida claimed this threw her schedule off for the entire day.

Personality: When Ida first entered New Start, she was compliant, even anxious to learn how to become independent. She impressed staff with her conversation, especially her ability to recount proper program philosophy. Initial evaluations by staff using the Blue Form identified her difficulties as money management, cooking, budgeting, and shopping. The staff soon discovered her most distinguishing and displeasing trait was that she required constant attention.

Ida's ability to manipulate adults into doing things for her was impressive. For example, a psychology student named Betty doing volunteer work at New Start was a woman in her mid-forties. Betty had advised Ida to call the beauty salon for an appointment, mentioning that it was good independent living behavior to set up appointments well in advance. With the telephone in its cradle at her side, Ida acted confused about which time she should take for her appointment, because the shop had offered her two times.

In her most helping and unobtrusive manner, Betty advised Ida to be flexible and take the noon time. Ida quickly countered saying she might have a schedule conflict. They parried back and forth for a few seconds until Ida agreed that she would be flexible, using Betty's term. With an appreciative look to Betty and an exhausted sigh of relief Ida fell back into the couch. Suddenly, she popped up and reminded Betty to call and secure the time!

Ida's powerful, dependent behavior was exhibited in full force during a grocery shopping observation seven months into the program. The trip became a series of overwrought disasters. First, she begged the observer to return to her apartment when she realized she had forgotten to make a shopping list. Once in her apartment, she was beset with more catastrophes: her mail bore bad news; she misplaced her wallet; and, finally, she began to feel an intense and tearful longing for her New Start counselor. Once her anxiety subsided, she found her wallet in her purse. Somewhat at ease, she retired to the bathroom, leaving the door ajar so she could maintain eye contact and conversation with the observer all the while.

Employment: Ida and Grace had no work history beyond sheltered workshops in which both had worked while enrolled in New Start. Following their graduations, they worked regularly as volunteers for Meals on Wheels, a charitable group which provides free meals to the elderly. When they were eventually told they would not be scheduled for work anymore, they were greatly disappointed.

Social Life: Grace turned out to be a terrific partner for Ida. She knew Ida's weekly schedule like her own because they shared the same activities. During the first couple of years on their own they did virtually everything together. Quiet, unassuming, attentive, and genuinely caring, Grace was only too happy to keep track of Ida's life, including her numerous complaints and ills.

In addition, while Ida was fighting with her mother, Grace's sister Rachel acted as a substitute for Ida's absent parent. Rachel visited the two roommates weekly, taking them to dinner, then shopping. Rachel also provided several comforts, such as furniture, for their home.

After several years passed and the women had become angry with each other, Grace made regular visits to a retarded man named Pete whom she had befriended. She complained that Ida would not allow her to visit Pete on her own, insisting on accompanying her. Ida's mother Verna encouraged Ida to tag along with Grace as she felt it did no harm.

Parental/Family Involvement: Ida said she was very close to her father. Her wall held the pictures that proved it: a recent photo of Ida and her father on a Carribbean cruise; Ida on the cruiseship deck in a girlish lavendar dress; another father and daughter photo in the Orient. She had traveled all over the world with her parents including trips to Scandinavia, China, Japan, and Europe. From the photos it seemed apparent that Ida valued her father's company and vice versa. Ida had an ambivalent relationship with her mother which at times was openly hostile.

Ida made it clear that she and her mother did not get along well. However, it was later confirmed that an important transition period during which Ida and her mother seldom communicated coincided with this investigation. Contrary to this author's impression, the absence of communication was unusual and atypical for them. Throughout a separate, later research project Ida and her mother maintained regular, weekly contact.

Grace and her sister Rachel were similarly mannered, tending to be quiet, gentle people who listened attentively and challenged rarely. They were polite in a dutiful, old-fashioned way which one observer viewed as emotional distance. Rachel was Grace's slightly detached caretaker. Grace assumed virtually the same role for Ida. Ida wanted someone to be involved in all aspects of her life, and Grace wanted someone to take care of. The match was so perfect at first, it was hard to accept that it eventually threatened to fail.

Summary: As companions, Ida and Grace were successful and, for the most part, independent program graduates. With Grace, Ida had managed to find a willing replacement for her caretaker father. Both women felt emotionally content in their independent lives.

However, the task of keeping Ida's life in balance may have exceeded Grace's capacity. Grace became angry enough to consider breaking away from Ida. Some felt that Grace would survive a separation much better than Ida. Perhaps Grace had outgrown her need to take care of Ida in order to feel competent, or more likely, Ida proved too difficult for Grace to tolerate. At the same time, Ida had not outgrown her need for a full-time caretaker.

Ida's first order of business upon entering New Start was to replace her father. New Start found a new parent for Ida in Grace. The same staff had previously paired Ida with Natalie who couldn't have been a worse choice. Natalie was a young, volatile Black woman who was extremely self-reliant. After two weeks with Ida's complaints and solicitations for assistance Natalie threatened to "tear her white nose off her face."

Ida and Grace were a platonic couple, initially committed as though they were marriage partners. Like the other two married couples, the Larsens and the Daltons, they were able to graduate from New Start with a chance. In this they probably achieved more as a pair than they could have on their own. The Larsens and Daltons shared many similarities both as individuals and couples although the Larsens' enmeshed relationship with cousin Roy distinguished them from the Daltons.

The partnership of Ida and Grace was significantly different than that of Walter and Stefan, the other platonic couple. By contrast, Ida and Grace exhibited many more dependent behaviors as a couple than did Walter and Stefan. The two young men were fiercely independent in spirit and practice while the two women nurtured a dependence on each other as long as possible. This difference became more apparent with each observation of Ida and Grace, and reinforced the idea that the pseudo-independents represented a final destination for some graduates in the pursuit of independent living.

Darlene Mears

Appearance: Darlene was a shy woman whose appearance had always been more youthful than her actual age. Her family was from Texas and she retained a West Texas drawl. She was like one of the hardy weeds that tumble across West Texas; unattractive, unadorned, frail-looking but resilient, with a tenacious will to survive that was easily overlooked by strangers.

The extent to which Darlene's clothes were out of date provided the most obvious cue that she was different. When first observed, her clothes had a funky, thrift store appeal which gave her a kooky '60s look. For instance, she would wear a round-collared, beige coat over a gold knit shift with sparkling gold buttons, and pointed black flats. Darlene looked poor. However, once she left New Start and got out on her own, she updated her style and wore contemporary clothes. She also restyled her hair and discovered makeup.

The difference, noted in a two-year followup, was startling to the observer:

> She looked different. She was slight as ever but less hunched over, and her hair showed the remains of a light blonde rinse about two months old. The most striking difference, however, was that she was clothed with a sense of current style. None of the old thrift store fare. She looked normal, not retarded. (author's field notes)

Personal Background: Observations of Darlene were among the most extensive within the sample. Her progress was observed as she participated in three consecutive training programs, each one designed to bring her closer to independent living. Motivated by necessity (her parents had informed her they would be unable to support her any longer), she quietly progressed toward her goal of living on her own.

The year prior to her enrollment in New Start, she was in an Independent Living Preparatory Class (ILPC) sponsored by a national fundraising organization for the handicapped. In this preliminary program she was introduced to the basic set of independent living skills; cooking, meal preparation, grocery shopping, laundry, transportation, and banking.

The ILPC training took place in a humble storefront which housed two large rooms, three small offices, and three very dedicated instructors who conducted the daily classes. Instruction began at the most fundamental level such as identifying units of food (pints, quarts) and money (pennies, nickels, dimes, quarters, and bills).

After several months of classroom instruction using facsimiles of store goods and currency, students were systematically dispatched to the community. Armed with tasks like "take the bus to the market and buy six items on a shopping list," the students practiced and mastered the basic skills. Darlene was a model student at ILPC.

Darlene entered New Start in April 1981 and graduated in March 1983. She had progressed through New Start in her characteristic manner; attracting little negative attention, completing all her tasks, and winning the staff's praise for her responsibility.

After graduation she moved into an apartment a few miles from the New Start office with her program roommate. The roommate's boyfriend moved in soon after. Darlene did not approve but did not protest. The roommate and boyfriend eventually moved out leaving Darlene in the apartment by herself.

Current Home Life: A follow-up visit two years later revealed that Darlene had stayed in the same apartment, which was located in a particularly unattractive area. At least in terms of dwellings, she had not shaken the appearance of poverty. The apartment was on a broad unmarked boulevard without an island or dividing strip. The area looked barren and bleak. In the immediate vicinity was a liquor store and an auto repair garage. All the buildings looked old and run down.

She and her roommate had furnished the entire apartment with used furniture, most of it in poor condition. Her living room was dark and small, with ample but shabby furnishings. She had a matching couch and love seat of brown, crushed velvet surrounding a coffee table. A side table with a lamp sat next to the couch. A beat-up color TV on a stand faced the seating area.

One lone painting adorned the walls. The couch and love seat had especially filthy arm rests from too many years of supporting greasy limbs. It initially appeared as though Darlene had made little progress in elevating the quality of her life. However, it soon became apparent that Darlene was not the same, and that her success could not be measured only by her dwelling.

Most importantly, she seemed to have grown comfortable with herself as a person. She spoke openly about her desire for a family, the importance of friendships to her, and her own sexuality. She said that she was unhappy about her current prospects for finding happiness in life, especially acquiring a mate. And she revealed she felt ignorant, though no longer innocent, about sex. Her candid disclosures were unexpected.

Darlene had also changed her approach to money; from being fearful and uncomfortable to being more relaxed and generous. She paid the entire rent herself and felt no pressure to take in a new roommate. New Start had helped her qualify for section 8 benefits.

Recently, she had purchased items which she once considered to be frivolous. These included her dog named Dorito ($25), a new bed (around $300), a color TV (also around $300), a clothes dryer (another $300), and a doll house ($75). Her mother helped her purchase the TV and bed acting as her advisor.

Her ability to save money from a monthly income of $600 was impressive, and a reminder of her miserly ways. Still, her most recent purchase (the bed) had nearly wiped out her savings. She said she only had $100 in savings and $400 in checking after paying her rent that month. As in the past, her mother provided no financial support.

Darlene had learned to use a calculator in managing her bankbooks. When she entered New Start she had already mastered cooking, cleaning and washing. Math, however, had always been tough. Now she opened her checkbook to show the neat and carefully written entries, a dollar sign preceding each one demonstrating her acquired competence.

Personality: Darlene was a shy individual, cooperative in attitude and behavior. She was the only member of the Pseudo-Independents who had not exhibited any signs of psychological disturbance or personality disorder. When she finally exited the system of social service agencies and programs in which she had participated for many years, she began to develop, or at least express, her own thoughts and wishes. This was a significant change in her personality.

Employment: Darlene had two jobs assisting disabled adults for a social service agency for non-ambulatory persons. She cleaned their apartments, accompanied them to the doctor, went shopping with them, etc.. She was paid to do for others what she had learned to do for herself in New Start. She had to quit working for a third client because he often made her travel out of her way, kept her too late, and threw tantrums.

She did not know exactly how much she got paid, but estimated it to be approximately $50 every two weeks. Her other source of income was SSI for which she received $504 monthly. Her paychecks went into her savings account while her SSI went into her checking account. That way she was able to save some money.

Social Life: At ILPC Darlene was very shy. Her social life consisted of TV and little else for many years. She apparently had no friends as she never mentioned outside activities. This had changed as her apartment held ample evidence of leisure-time diversions.

In her sunny kitchen stood an easel with a canvas and paints spread on newspaper over the kitchen table. She was working on a paint-by-numbers picture of a sailing ship. She had purchased a new color TV last year, which had been stolen one Sunday while she was at church. She had acquired a pet dog for $25 (which she had first cleared with the landlord) named Dorito. Dorito sat in Darlene's lap where he received lots of hugging and petting.

Darlene had defeated her isolation with several new activities; artwork, a pet, and a friendship with the single mother of two who lived upstairs. By Darlene's account, the relationship with her neighbor was both the most rewarding and the most taxing.

Darlene enjoyed a mutually exploitative friendship with her. The young mother wanted a cheap babysitter on the weekends, and Darlene wanted a family. Darlene frequently babysat the children, often overnight. Sometimes she was paid, sometimes not. The mother would counsel Darlene about what to value in a relationship with a man. If you can't have love then at least get material goods, she advised. As a result, Darlene seemed to have developed her own hard-boiled attitude about the single lifestyle. She shared this perspective in comments she made about families, love, and sex. Darlene said:

> I can't find any nice guys. Seems all they want is sex, especially the younger ones, the teenagers. I met a guy like that who only wanted sex. I don't mind sex. It's okay some of the time, but sometimes I'd like to go out, too. My penis, I mean my thing, is too small and it hurts me when they put their penis in. And they won't stop when I ask them.

She practiced birth control (the pill) but experienced side effects. Her gynecologist switched her from one device to another several times. She did not menstruate very often which caused her and her social workers great concern. Apparently, Darlene had been sexually active with several young men.

Darlene reinforced her friendship with her neighbor's oldest daughter by purchasing a $75 doll house kit for the girl which the two were in the process of assembling. The doll house was in Darlene's back bedroom along with the new clothes dryer. She also had a pet bird in the room, in a cage. Darlene had purchased the doll house for the girl's Christmas present but gave it to her a couple of months early. The girl had already bought several pieces of furniture for the house. They planned to finish it together with paint and wallpaper.

Parental/Family Involvement: Darlene's parents (Mr. and Mrs. Schatz) seemed relatively uninvolved. Unlike most of the parents of other sample members, the Schatzes maintained a very low profile with the various agencies involved in her progress.

Mrs. Schatz was Darlene's primary, if marginal, support person. She provided help in the form of furniture and clothing hand-me-downs, and made an occasional small gift of cash. When Darlene attended ILPC she was outfitted by her mother. ILPC staff commented that although Darlene's clothes were clean and presentable they were very outdated, as though they had been carefully picked off the racks at the Salvation Army or Goodwill stores.

Darlene's quiet awkwardness extended to her attitude toward money. She never seemed to have much, but when she did, she was quite uncomfortable. Her mother seemed to hold the same poverty-bred attitude.

For example, Darlene's mother wanted to provide some financial support to help Darlene move into the New Start apartment. She gave Darlene $60 to purchase towels and sheets. Darlene was unusually concerned throughout the shopping trip, especially over a purse she had bought on impulse for seven dollars. She worried that she had wasted the money and would have to face her mother's disapproval. The purse was not on her shopping list; it was something extra, a treat.

Summary: Darlene greatly reduced her stigma of poverty when she moved into her own place. Her neighborhood and her furniture suggested little growth, but her statements about herself, her appearance, her friendship with her neighbor, her work as a companion, and her comfort with money indicated that she was making progress in her life. Her wishes for a life of even greater fulfillment were her greatest luxury.

Nevertheless, Darlene had no plans for improving her situation, and her present state of harmony seemed dependent on her neighbor's presence. Her success was like a world of small pleasures, each of which she enjoyed immensely.

Darlene seemed to have no set future. She also had no special benefactor to help her in crises or to guide her toward a goal. The upstairs neighbor's primary commitment to Darlene was as a convenient companion. Francis Larsen's cousin Roy, and Grace's sister Rachel, provided far more assistance, by comparison. Darlene was truly on her own, in that she had no one to depend on but herself.

On the other hand, Darlene had ambitions which exceeded those of Ida and Grace, and at least paralleled those of the Larsens. She was financially independent, and apparently well-established with the welfare system. She hadn't suffered any problems with SSI and enjoyed the benefits of Section 8 rent assistance (monetary aid for qualified renters). Darlene was functioning independently and with reasonable happiness in the present, yet her station in life seemed so vulnerable to upheaval that one could only wonder how long it would last.

Aileen Karnan

Appearance: Aileen was a short, plump, sleepy-eyed young woman who would have been easily missed in a group. Her appearance was unremarkable and, in this sense, she did not look retarded or handicapped. Her manner, speech, and nervous behavior, however, revealed her to be a very insecure, preoccupied, and, at times, bizarre person.

Personal Background: Aileen was observed on six separate occasions during her enrollment in New Start. She was 34 years old when she graduated. Coincidentally, the observer had met and chatted with Aileen's parents a few times at the New Start office. They made it clear that they wished to be more involved in the program than it seemed able to tolerate. A follow-up phone interview was conducted with Aileen one year after she graduated from the New Start program. Her SDD worker also provided information on her progress as a participant and graduate of the New Start program.

New Start placed Aileen in a one-bedroom apartment with a wheelchair-bound, handicapped woman about her age who had been with New Start for one year. Since the roommate held seniority, Aileen slept in the living room. The observer noted that the place was generally unkempt and run down. Aileen was unhappy with the roommate match.

Assessment of her skills at entry showed she was weak in all the standard areas of cooking, grocery shopping, budgeting, and housekeeping. Observations confirmed these assessments. For example, at the checkout line in the market she could not provide proper bill denominations. At the bank, she was unable to respond to the teller's queries about how she wanted her money. She was unable to calculate correct change on several occasions in several settings.

Observations of her cooking showed she had low skill levels in basic tasks. For example, she was scheduled to be observed preparing lamb chops. When the observer arrived she realized that she had forgotten to defrost the meat. She quickly tried to assemble a substitute dinner of instant soup and white bread-with-a-slice-of-bologna sandwich.

This stood in contrast to the confidence she demonstrated in doing laundry, which was also her chore when she lived with her parents in New York. She had prepared by doing most of the laundry the night before. She had purposely just left enough unwashed to demonstrate her skill. She washed and dried the clothes then neatly folded them and put them away. Unlike her performances in the other tasks, she was calm and anxiety-free.

Current Home Life: When Aileen was interviewed almost a year and a half after her graduation from New Start, her demeanor had changed noticably.

She was indifferent to the observer and resisted his invitation to be interviewed. When she agreed to talk, it was on the spur of the moment. She spoke once for 40 minutes then told the observer she was finished. She made no pretense about closing the interview. She stated she had simply lost interest in talking about herself any longer.

During the interview, she was polite and seemed genuine in her responses. Although she did not exhibit her previous need to please others, the observer learned that much of the relationship with her parents, at least in terms of services they provided, was still intact.

She still depended on them for much support. They had found her an apartment in Santa Monica which she shared with a roommate. New Start had helped her qualify for Section 8 assistance so her monthly rent was halved, to $268. Her parents gave her $400 to $500 monthly to cover expenses. The money was deposited directly into her savings account. She dined with them weekly at her favorite delicatessen.

She did not use checks but she did have a savings account. She admitted that she still could not manage a checking account. She paid her rent with money orders (the New Start method), and preferred to carry about $40 in cash with her (another New Start recommendation). She took pride in her ability to use the bus system well enough to go to her psychiatrist appointment every two weeks in Beverly Hills. Other common bus excursions included traveling to a nearby drug store for shopping, or to her mother's home for a drop-in visit.

Personality: Aileen's SDD worker believed Aileen needed to accomplish individuation, a developmental task of separating from the parent and forming a separate identity. The SDD worker identified Aileen's relationship with her parents as her primary obstacle.

Aileen offered no resistance to entering New Start. As several sources have noted, she was anxious to please others around her, especially her parents. Observation notes repeatedly cite how much she seemed to value the attention of the observer. She apologized repeatedly for imposing on others' time.

She was described as overcooperative, extremely anxious, self-conscious, giggling constantly, too nervous to perform simple tasks, babbling and rambling in her speech, and so ill at ease with herself that the observer also felt terribly uncomfortable in her presence.

Employment: Aileen participated in none of the standard activities that other subjects typically substituted for a competitive job; no volunteer work or sheltered workshop.

Social Life: Apparently, she had not developed much of a social life beyond the routine excursions with her parents. She identified her friends as fellow New Start grads Sally Redland (to be discussed under the Failures) and Jessica (unknown to the observer). She said that Sally seldom had time for her. When interviewed Sally described Aileen as "too dorky." Aileen either failed to acknowledge this shabby treatment or simply did not realize she was being brushed off.

Parental/Family Involvement: Aileen's parents were involved to the point of becoming enmeshed with her training program. They spent much of their time monitoring her program plan. The Karnans moved from New York City in order to enroll Aileen in the New Start program. It was their first attempt to place their beloved daughter outside their home. They were retired educators, both holding advanced academic degrees.

Their sheltering of Aileen all her life was evidenced by her poor social skills and apparent naivete concerning common social behaviors. The manner in which they oversaw New Start activities had a compulsive and suspicious quality which the Karnans explained as professional curiosity. Nevertheless, the New Start staff felt pressured by their presence. They described Aileen's parents as meddlesome and oppressive. Aileen's SDD worker described the effect:

> The Karnans were very involved with New Start. They made their presence known and frequently donated money or needed items to New Start. When they expressed dissatisfaction regarding the program or Aileen's lack of progress, they were listened to and adjustments or changes were put into effect. The Karnans had an overwhelming need for the program to be what it was not, a vehicle of transformation for their daughter. It was far easier to place blame on the program than on the cognitive and emotional deficits exhibited by their daughter...

The New Start staff were aware of the consistent overinvolvement of Aileen's parents in her life, but failed to confront them and, instead, complained heartily to other staff about their constant meddling. The SDD worker argued that this kind of support was more a liability than an asset and was a way in which the parents denied their daughter's handicap.

Prior to New Start, and even while she was enrolled in the program, the Karnans provided for Aileen's finances, food, clothing, and entertainment. Their powerful axis of support proved too strong for New Start to supplant. Almost two years after graduation from New Start, the interaction between Aileen and her parents had, by Aileen's report, not changed substantially.

Summary: In retrospect, Aileen stated that New Start did not help her very much, the counselors were not very nice and were often too busy for her. Her SDD worker commented that Aileen did not fit the profile of new enrollees at New Start. She pointed out that Aileen was accepted into the program without any prior formal training in independent living skills. This placed Aileen at a disadvantage in relation to her peers and, in the worker's opinion, impeded Aileen's ability to separate from her parents.

The three most important consequences of her New Start experience seemed to have been finding an apartment to live in on her own in a safe and attractive part of town; being able to maintain her supportive links with her parents which, in turn, allowed her to evade the possible negative consequences of her deficient skills in money management and food planning; and building up her self-esteem by receiving a certificate of independence from New Start.

When interviewed in the follow-up phone conversation, Aileen felt she was independent and claimed she was enjoying life in her own apartment. She defined being independent as trying to do her own thing. Aileen's lifestyle strongly resembled that of Ida and Grace. All three women felt independent and lived on their own. Each maintained important lines of support with their family members. The greatest difference was that Ida and Grace provided a social life for each other which extended beyond their families. According to Aileen and her SDD worker she was almost exclusively dependent on her parents for her entertainment and social activity.

The Karnans' involvement in their daughter's life was virtually ubiquitous, and certainly one of the most enmeshed for the sample subjects discussed to this point. Aileen's SDD worker felt this involvement was like a time-bomb ready to go off. She feared that once Aileen was left truly alone in her apartment the deficits in her New Start training would become manifest.

June LePoap

Appearance: Her receding chin and large, wide open eyes were set on a face which seemed oversized for her petite frame. She preferred to wear her bleached blonde hair in a modified beehive which fit her southeastern, country-bred roots. The initial cues that she was retarded were quickly forgotten once she displayed her gracious social skills and casual demeanor. Her speech flowed easily, with a sincerity that made it easy to relax under the special charms of southern hospitality.

June seamlessly integrated so many conflicting qualities in her life that she was, in an aggregate way, the quintessential example of the Pseudo-Independent program graduate. She presented a very convincing appearance of independent competence which stood in marked contrast to her obviously camouflaged dependencies.

Personal Background: The observer met with June after she had graduated New Start, but had known of her by reputation in the program. At New Start, her roommate was a wheelchair-bound woman for whom June was the caretaker. June had also remained at New Start for 36 months, longer than any other participant. Her regional center worker provided much information regarding June's experiences in becoming independent.

June was from Indiana and Kentucky. Her conversation was laden with racial prejudice and conservative values about women and family. Her self-image as a functional and successful human being was consistent with her views. For example, she believed she was skilled at mothering others, which she stated was a valuable and traditional role for women. She was against women's liberation. She made several references to having been a mother figure to her three grown children, her peers at New Start and her neighbors in her current residence, a United Cerebral Palsy (UCP) home.

She had been dependent on others all her life yet her greatest strength was her own ability to make others depend on her. She was admitted into her new residence on the strength of these skills. June learned her homemaking and caretaking skills, first as an adolescent surrogate mother, and then as a young mother. June dropped out of school to take care of the household when her mother died. Leaving school was probably a welcome opportunity for June, as she recalled her school experiences with regret. She described herself as a "slow reader" who was never placed in any special class.

She met her future husband, James LePoap (also a "slow reader") after leaving high school. They married (she was 18 years old) and moved to Kentucky. Several years later they moved to California. June bore three children; two boys, 23 and 20 years old at the time of our interview, and a daughter, who was 24 years old. Once in California she separated from her husband and her family. She was less revealing on this point although she said enough to allow the observer to infer that he physically abused her. When she recalled this stressful time in her life, she made several references to the Bible in an effort to close the subject on a good note. Her SDD worker confirmed that June had endured several physically abusive relationships in her lifetime, including her first marriage. Following the failure of that marriage, June moved in with her sister who completely supported her. In return, June took care of the housekeeping. During her stay with her sister she qualified for SSI which she needed to enter New Start.

Current Home Life: Being admitted as a resident in the UCP facility was competitive and June had numerous interviews before being accepted. She was the only resident without cerebral palsy. She described herself as a staff person. One of her duties was to prepare group meals several times a week.

The home was a new two-story apartment building a few miles from the beach, adjacent to a concrete water channel at the end of a quiet residential block. Two thirds of the rent on the 16 new apartments was paid for by Section 8 funds, and one third by the residents. The building's backyard was a lovely, landscaped, grassy space where residents could sit in the sun. All the first floor apartments had sliding doors that opened onto the yard. It was the nicest group home for the handicapped the observer had ever seen.

June had acquired this particular apartment for herself. Only the live-in residential supervisor, with her husband and young child, had a nicer living space. June's one-bedroom, upstairs flat faced the ocean and river. Within only 600 square feet, she had a separate kitchen and living area with a spacious bathroom, which was equipped for use by the handicapped. She had decorated her apartment very nicely, and it was in pristine condition. Her homemaking skills were impressive judging by the attention she had obviously paid to developing a thematic sense to her decor; that of breezy, sunshine-filled Southern California in colors of yellow, orange and white.

Personality: She fit the profile for the battered wife: few personal resources;

low self-esteem; history of violence and abuse; alcoholism; abandonment by parents at an early age; and little insight. Her SDD worker noted that June did not accept this image of herself. June also did not believe that having her sister handle all her finances meant she was less than independent. Instead, she felt that as long as the SSI check was in her name, like the apartment, she was pulling her own weight.

She compensated for most of her deficits with her substantial and impressive charm. Of course, this had limited, short-term benefit.

Employment: She had never worked competitively in her life. The only income she ever received in her name was from SSI.

Social Life: June's twin sister, Sissy, traveled to Los Angeles from Palm Springs once a week for her job, visiting June on the way home. At this time she gave June $50 for weekly expenses and took her shopping for food and other essentials. Sissy often stayed overnight.

The caseworker confirmed that June's current amorous relationship was an abusive one. There had been more than one episode of drunken fighting between the two in her apartment which had placed her status in jeopardy at the UCP home. June described the relationship as a "romantic involvement with a male friend."

Her primary social interactions were accomplished in her role as mother to the UCP residents. This had been a trend throughout her life.

Parental/Family Involvement: June's twin sister, Sissy, lived in Palm Springs, worked for a Los Angeles aviation firm, and was a Christian singer in her free time. By June's account, Sissy had devoted much of her life to June's welfare and had been instrumental in getting June into the New Start program.

June was quite dependent on her sister, especially for money. June's rent was $101 per month; she received an $84 credit monthly for her weekly duties preparing meals. She found checkbooks too confusing. With her sister's help, she felt she could get along without one.

Her SSI check was deposited directly into Sissy's Palm Springs bank account. In a defensive manner, June volunteered that Sissy would bring more money than the weekly $50 if June so wished. To support her point she offered the following explanation. "I deal with cash. I can make change. Not needing Sissy's financial assistance anymore makes me feel independent."

Summary: Despite her obvious dependencies on her sister and the protected environment of the UCP home, June believed she was independent, especially since she had graduated New Start and moved to her new home as a quasi-staff member.

In the UCP home June had found a shelter where she could safely make her place, becoming a part of the staff in a limited capacity, and feeling her life held value to herself and others. For June, as for many battered women, such an outcome would be considered a significant success.

June was a divorced mother whose children had grown up apart from her. She was untrained in any vocation and unwilling to compete for a job.

She found a niche where she could feel good about herself and utilize her lifelong skill: homemaking.

SECTION SUMMARY:
THE PSEUDO-INDEPENDENTS

The first subjects discussed, the Larsens, were a couple who had unwillingly relinquished their financial independence, albeit without much of a struggle, to a relative, cousin Roy. The cousin had total control of their financial decisions. The Larsens had a social life of their own (even though they were dissatisfied with it), they lived in their own apartment in the normal community, and one of them held a regular job, even though he obtained it through nepotism.

The last subject discussed in the group was June LePoap who, in contrast to the Larsens, happily placed control of her finances with her sister, who was also her primary helper. June had an active, though troubled, social life, and lived in a sheltered facility where she enjoyed staff status.

Somewhere between these extremes were the platonically paired women in their fifties, Ida and Grace, who had been sheltered all but the last three or four years of their fully mature lives. Together they had learned to live on their own in the community without the constant supervision of their parents or family helpers. However, Ida's extreme psychological dependency brought so much tension to their partnership that their separation seemed imminent. Such an event was viewed as potentially beneficial to Grace, but devastating to Ida. In any event, they required and expected ongoing support from several sources.

Darlene and Aileen, two single and similarly shy women, presented markedly different cases of parental involvement and social adjustment (one with excessively involved parents and the other with a minimally involved parent). Darlene was compliant while Aileen was rebellious and highly manipulative. Neither enjoyed friendships at New Start.

Once out of the program Darlene was able to initiate a relationship with her neighbor's family. Aileen remained extremely enmeshed with her mother and father. Darlene was the sole subject in this group who had complete control of her own finances.

For every Pseudo-Independent subject the extent of parental, or familial, involvement was much greater than with the Independents. Francis, the only competitively employed subject in this group, had his income controlled by the same cousin who employed him in such an autocratic manner that made the financial control exercised by Janice's mother seem comparatively benign.

Another criterion which seemed to differentiate these seven subjects from the Independents was the presence of psychosocial pathology in their lives. Psychological issues within this group were also more prominent. They included alcoholism (Francis Larsen and June LePoap), physical abuse (June), schizo-affective behavior (Aileen), immaturity (Kristy Larsen), and a probable personality disorder (Ida). Within the group, Darlene and Grace were the only two subjects without prominent psychological problems.

Yet, all the subjects in this group graduated from New Start and were able to live on their own, having successfully freed themselves from living with their natural families. All had secured stable incomes including whatever they received from their parents or other relatives. Their patchworks of trust funds, parental gifts, SSI, sheltered workshop pay, state and federal health coverage, and state or county aid to renters (e.g., Section 8 funds) kept them in the community and out of their parents' or other board and care homes. Their levels and sources of income most resembled those of retirees or the physically disabled.

The Pseudo-Independents had not clearly succeeded in their efforts to move into the community and live independently. They had not failed, either. They had not achieved the levels of independence which were found in the lives of the preceding five subjects, all of whom worked (except one), controlled the extent of the contact with their parent/helper, and managed their own finances (except one). The Pseudo-Independent subjects were far more likely to retain some ongoing contact with a formal agency; whether it was New Start, SDD, or UCP.

Unlike the Independents, most of the Pseudo-Independents (except possibly Darlene and the Larsens) did not seek to strive further. Their success was a new kind, requiring this investigator to rethink his concept of success and independence in terms of their actual lives. The Pseudo-Independents had reached their pinnacles of success. They had carefully constructed their worlds: positioning their helpers, for the most part, in a positive if dependent relationship; securing sources of income which were marginal and fixed, yet sufficient for their reduced living standards; and making living arrangements which were stable, selected for convenience over luxury. They had acquired possessions which provided entertainment and gave them a sense of stature. They had put together daily routines or friendships which enabled them to feel valuable to others. They had reached their destinations in independent living.

Pseudo-Independents were both independent and dependent, living with contradictions that perplexed the observer. From a conservative and, perhaps, cynical perspective, it could be argued that these subjects had achieved all that could be justifiably expected from them given that they graduated from a program which was generally disorganized and poorly administered.

Like their program, the Pseudo-Independents maintained a facade of independence belied by the evidence, yet they maintained that they felt independent. To paraphrase some of them, independence meant being self-governing, not being subject to control by others, not having to rely on others, not being affiliated with a larger controlling organization, feeling free, and being absent from constraint. Observations revealed that their own definitions of independence were incompatible with their lives.

Chapter 6

The
Failures

The final three subjects were strikingly similar in several ways; each was younger than 30, exceptionally articulate, quite normal in appearance, had a generally engaging personality, and kept current with the cultural trends and themes of their generation. None were working when they graduated from New Start. Each disdained sheltered workshops almost as much as they disliked the label of mental retardation. As with the Pseudo-Independents, there was evidence that psychopathology impeded their abilities to live independently. Additionally, their psychological issues seemed to stem in part from labeling; they were all badly stigmatized by the nature of their handicap.

Ernie Reiss

Appearance: Ernie was 19 years old when he entered New Start. He had sandy hair and a slouched posture. He was tall and lanky-framed.

Despite his gentle, carefree nature, first impressions of Ernie were often based on the greasy, clumpy hair which hung in his eyes; his multi-hued jeans painted by skin oils; and the stinky-sweet odor that marked his living space. His voice struggled to break through his occluded nostrils. With all these repelling distractions, it was difficult to recognize his more charming traits such as his softspoken manner, unexpectedly quick mind, and ready sense of humor.

Personal Background: Ernie had the second highest intelligence test scores of the entire sample. He had material resources that exceeded those of all but one subject. He passed through the New Start program unremarkably, after which he returned to the home he had lived in for most of his life. On his own, unemployed, and with virtually no friends or daily routine, his life and his home quickly fell into disrepair.

Ernie graduated from New Start in 26 months. His stay in the program was quiet and generally uneventful, as had been his life until his mother's sudden death from an aneurism which prompted his entry into the program. Ernie's grandmother was quickly moved into the home by his divorced father until Ernie was placed in New Start six weeks later. Ernie felt coerced and agreed to go on one condition; that he be allowed to return to his home once he completed the program.

Current Home Life: The fact that Ernie quit his only job because the work was too dirty (handling newspapers) was somewhat ironic in that his personal hygiene was so awful. His unwashed body and clothes were visibly grimy:

> We enter his apartment and the stink is overwhelming. The place smells like a month's worth of sweat and dirty laundry. It is a pigsty. Newspapers are strewn everywhere. Pieces of bread lay about the floor. His dirty underpants are on the carpet. (author's field notes).

Ernie had equally poor dietary practices. He disliked brushing his teeth. He had youthful energy and fairly good health, except for the superficial infections and sores which resulted from his horrid diet. He stated that when his mother fed him he never got the painful sores but now that he was feeding himself he got them quite often. He believed that his reluctance to eat vegetables and leafy greens was the cause.

During one observation he walked about the room with a bottle of Chloraseptic, spraying the interior of his mouth with a shot or two every few minutes as we talked. When he did not eat at home he went out to Pioneer Chicken. When he cooked it was usually spaghetti with sauce from a jar, or Shake 'N Bake chicken.

For the 26 months Ernie spent in New Start, he was roommates with a young man named Bill, who was diagnosed as schizophrenic. The match could hardly have been worse. Ernie needed to develop social skills. A roommate with a strong personality and decent social skills would have been an appropriate choice. Ernie needed to replace his mother who had to this point provided for all his social and emotional needs. Instead, he was placed with a schizophrenic, whose behavior was isolative and bizarre.

The match provided no opportunity for Ernie to grow as an adult. On the other hand, Bill received no challenge to behave appropriately from the soft-spoken, inexperienced Ernie. From a behavior management perspective, the staff had a trouble-free apartment. But, in terms of the ability of two participants to promote growth in each other, the pairing of Ernie and Bill was a complete failure.

Although Bill was compulsive and Ernie was undisciplined the two never clashed. Bill was never known to have complained about Ernie's appalling personal hygiene or housekeeping. Bill's room stood in stark, pristine contrast to Ernie's chaotic world which began immediately outside Bill's door. Bill's room was neat and ordered, while the living room and hall were strewn with newspapers, articles of clothing, fast food wrappings and other trash. Bill spent most of his time in his room, seldom emerging except to prepare food. Ernie confided that they never went out together, and stated that he would have preferred a roommate with whom he could go places. They only interacted in the kitchen. They were both bad cooks with equally sloppy techniques. Ernie's attempt to cook a meat loaf was typically unsanitary as well as uninformed:

Ernie is cooking Southern Meat Loaf tonight. He has lifted the recipe from a book he checked out at the public library. The book is six months overdue. He is very literal about the recipe so that when it says to add four slices of bread he tosses in four whole slices!! I suggest he break them into pieces. . .He washed his hands. . .(which) he immediately dirties by crawling around on the filthy floor searching for a utensil. He wipes them off on his jeans which are also filthy, as usual. In preparing the meat loaf he selects his only pan which is more suitable for lasagna. But it is his only pan. . .Ernie places all the ingredients on the counter and opens all the cans first. He points out to me that the recipe calls for 1.5 pounds of beef and he has only 1.1 pounds. He is specific about the decimals. He opens the refrigerator to remove the meat and a powerful stench fills the room. He reaches for spices and I notice the army of ants moving on the cupboard in a wave. After realizing that the pan is in fact much too large, he places all in a bowl and pops it in the oven. (author's field notes).

Ernie's problems with meal preparation and diet began at the market. At the grocery store he tried to limit his spending to $20, as suggested by New Start staff. This limit was intended to curb the resident's impulse buying. It had no impact on food selection, which was one of Ernie's problems. On one trip to the market he purchased bread and jam, cereal, cookies, apple juice, ice cream, frozen peas and corn, bologna, hot dogs, grapes, and bananas. He defended his purchase of hot dogs by stating, "you got to have some meat." His guidelines seemed to be to buy the cheapest product in the smallest amount, paying no attention to unit pricing.

New Start emphasized making a grocery list, using a calculator to track expenses, clipping coupons, choosing fresh foods, attending to unit pricing, and checking expiration dates. Of these techniques, Ernie focused on staying within his budget using a calculator, which appealed to his fondness for math. This permitted him to apply a skill he already possessed, but did nothing to improve his food selection or nutritional health. During another shopping trip he used his calculator, but forgot to make a list or bring coupons.

Along with selecting and preparing food, Ernie had also made little progress while at New Start in managing his finances. He received no SSI, had two savings accounts, and no checking account. Nearly four years after graduating, his skills were still woefully inadequate in these areas, as well as in housekeeping.

Eighteen months after graduating from New Start, Ernie had moved back into his mother's former home. It was a modest two-bedroom, one-bath house in a middle class neighborhood, that looked shabbier than his neighbors' homes. His lawn was overgrown and the paint was peeling:

The back yard was absurdly overgrown and untamed. In the near corner rested an electric mower, its cord disappearing into the brush. The yard was criss-crossed with random trails of mowed grass. He told me that he had encountered much difficulty mowing the lawn as the grass was so thick the blades clogged up every 15 minutes forcing the motor to quit. He would then shut the machine off and wait for the grass to dry, then shake it out. When he felt so inclined he would then go at it for another 15 minutes. (author's field notes).

Christmas lights surrounded the facade even though the season was four weeks past. All the shades were drawn, he explained, to fight the heat. The inside was as messy as his New Start apartment had been. There was the familiar smell of dirty laundry and decaying food, but not as strong as in his former apartment. He had been living alone for six months after having had a roommate for a year. He immediately said he was lonely and had been disappointed that his year-long roommate had been very isolative, retiring to his bedroom all the time.

Employment: According to Ernie all he needed to do was get a job. He clung to this belief throughout the observations, during and after New Start even though he had little comprehension of the work world. He believed that if he could only find a job "everything else would fall into place."

Ernie did find one job immediately after graduating from New Start, working with a newspaper. After six months he quit "because it was too dirty," making sure not to tell his father and stepmother for a few months.

Social Life: He was socially isolated, being both friendless and having interests that were solitary in nature. He was skilled in math, formal organizational schemes, and tedious record-keeping; however, his personal grooming was so poor that he was seldom recognized for his special talents.

Ernie had found a way to utilize his intellectual talents tracking weather data as a hobby. He diligently kept a record of daily temperatures in cities around the nation by creating a simple database which he could cross reference by date and location. At first, he kept the charts religiously, taking pleasure and pride in being able to discuss the seasonal changes as well as annual differences for any region of the country. He could claim with authority whether or not the current temperatures were typical or unusual for the season which made for fascinating conversation.

Ernie's hobby demonstrated two important skills: he could organize and maintain detailed records with good reliability—an attractive work skill; and he could converse easily when he felt he was knowledgable—an important social skill. Unfortunately, he and New Start were unable to apply these skills in any other setting, especially with regard to work or making friends.

Parental/Family Involvement: He was deeply saddened by his mother's sudden death. Their relationship was very close, which had probably been to his disadvantage. She either looked the other way when it came to his personal hygiene, or else she took care of all the tasks which resulted in a clean appearance; such as washing his clothes, picking up his room, and making sure he changed his clothes daily. It seemed likely that she was his only friend.

Ernie had remained in contact with New Start after graduation. At that time, New Start was in considerable organizational disarray. The follow-up program was the most intact service still offered. Yet, since leaving New Start, Ernie had been assigned four different counselors, who visited him irregularly. He recognized that he still needed help with his cooking, acknowledging that he ate "a lot of TV dinners."

His father had set up a simple system intended to handle all of Ernie's financial needs, as well as to avoid simple mistakes. The system featured two separate accounts, and most of the bill paying was handled by his father. From one savings account, Ernie's father gave him $80 weekly to take care of his personal and incidental expenses. His father also made the monthly house payment of $800 from this account.

The other savings account was to be used for emergencies only. Even though the system may have seemed relatively fail-safe to the father, it confused his son. When Ernie burned out the clutch in his car, he wrote the check out of the monthly expenses account instead of the emergency account, overdrawing it, and invoking penalty fees.

The particular kinds of support which Ernie received from his parents did not foster personal growth. By doing everything for him in the areas of housekeeping and socialization, his mother had made it unnecessary for Ernie to develop self-reliance in these areas. By keeping total control of Ernie's financial affairs, his father and stepmother had allowed Ernie to remain dependent on them for his livelihood. There was genuine reason to be concerned for how Ernie would manage once his father moved away.

Summary: Ernie appeared to have achieved a high level of success. He seemed to have it all: a house he owned; a car to drive that was paid for; a roommate to share expenses; an inheritance to supplement income; and a certificate that said he was ready to live independently. Ernie should have been a major success story for New Start. He had the ability to learn the necessary skills when capably motivated. For example, when his father bought him a small car as a New Start graduation gift, he took lessons, passed the test, and started driving.

Still, he had no social life and little prospect for any. He felt as though he were broke and saw little prospect for generating his own income. Ernie knew what changes he wanted to take place in his life, but expected to achieve none until he landed a job. He listed what he expected to achieve once he found work; his personal blueprint for success:

1. go out socially and feel less lonely
2. pay the entire monthly house note on his own
3. feel less depressed and dependent on his father
4. keep a cleaner home
5. eat better
6. not have money management problems

Forty-four months after entering New Start Ernie understood exactly what he was lacking in his life. He did not find anyone, such as his mother, father, or a New Start counselor, who could help him develop a program plan that might help him meet his needs.

An SDD worker familiar with his case wrote the following about Ernie:

> Ernie seems to just float along without any realistic goals established...I can't help but wonder if Ernie would not have fared better had the New Start program been more behaviorally oriented. It might have been great to have Ernie on a point system so that he could tap into his mathematical abilities and tally up his points earned daily in each category. It could be 'doubly reinforcing;' he would earn points and praise for tasks well done and could also be rewarded for his organizational skills. There is the potential for change in this young man.

The worker's idea for instituting a behavior modification regimen such as a token economy might have produced results with Ernie. However, such a plan required more attention, knowledge, and organization than New Start seemed able to offer. The placement of Ernie with the schizophrenic Bill represented a low point in the program's failure to consider the importance of interpersonal, psychological issues in fomenting success.

Sally Redland

Appearance: Sally was a 31-year-old female who easily passed for a high school student. She had a short, wiry frame, curly brown hair, and was normal looking.

Personal Background: Sally was quite verbal and conversed easily, especially if the subject concerned one of her main preoccupations: rock-and-roll music, the Rolling Stones rock band, cruising malls, or meeting boys. These fixtures of female teen subculture were Sally's cultural reference points.

When she entered New Start she was already an accomplished cook, kept an exceptionally neat home and kitchen, knew how to shop for all kinds of goods, but did not handle her money on her own. During her time in the program, however, she demonstrated the ability to handle her own money. She was observed making basic bank transactions, with only one minor error. When she lived at home, she performed all these tasks except for banking which her mother handled.

Sally graduated from New Start after two years in the program. To her dissatisfaction, one year later, she had moved back into her parents' apartment. She stated she felt she was more advanced at the time she graduated but had just gone backward since then, which she attributed to being "too close" to her family.

Current Home Life: Sally was observed preparing a meal of spaghetti and meatballs. She prepared the sauce from cans of tomato paste and sauce, ground beef, and vegetables. She attributed her mastery of this dish to having watched and helped her mother prepare it so often. She was also observed six weeks later shopping at the market for the standby spaghetti and meat-balls. She moved through the market swiftly, collecting all the items on her list in a systematic and routine manner. Once again, she acknowledged that she had learned to shop in the company of her mother.

However, since Sally had returned home she had ceased to practice her independent living skills, even those which she had mastered prior to New Start. She did not bank, shop for groceries, pay her bills, budget her weekly expenses, or cook her daily meals. Her only duty was to clean the house once a week on Thursday or Friday morning. She was not sure what she had in savings, only acknowledging that she "tried to save."

She felt trapped at home. Her plan for escaping was a familiar one; to get some job training and move out on her own. For example, she had heard of job training run by Children's Foundation which served the needs of the handicapped. It sounded hopeful except for one thing; she was repelled at the prospect of being in the company of "more program people."

Personality: Sally's SDD worker wrote that three factors were central to her personality makeup: denial of her handicap; an abnormal, symbiotic rela-tionship with her mother; and deep ambivalence about living independently.

Sally and her mother adhered to the belief that Sally was not retarded but rather that she had an "emotional problem." Sally was angry about "her role as retarded" and made a point of letting the observer know she was okay and that nothing was wrong with her. Her mother consistently denied to Sally and to others that her daughter was cognitively limited even though she had spent her entire public school career in special classes. Her SDD worker wrote that Sally learned to present herself apologetically from a lifetime of having to explain that she was not what she seemed; e.g., in special classes but not retarded like her classmates.

The worker wrote that as long as Sally lived with her mother she would play the part of the "obedient child complying with her mother's inappropri-ate, patronizing demands." These demands included having an evening cur-few hour, and having her behavior closely monitored by her mother.

The worker believed Sally realized that living independently held an in-herent threat to her self-image of being not retarded. "Should Sally leave the safety of her mother's home," he wrote, "she could fail and it would then be verified for all the world to see that she is truly retarded."

Sally had, according to her worker, "overwhelming anxieties about her abilities and her lack of them." To no surprise, demands for performance usually produced great anxiety in Sally. She tended to avoid performing tasks in which she was less than supremely confident. When she failed to perform at less than a flawless level she personally suffered. During a shopping trip she had problems counting change at the register. Her bill was $21.09 for which she gave the checker a $20 bill. When the checker said she needed more money Sally was visibly flustered and gave her a $10 bill even though she had several ones in her hand. Afterward Sally was quite angry with herself for "messing up." Her worker believed that Sally's reticence to attempt to master new tasks was an expression of her own confusion about herself.

Employment: Sally maintained that working in a rock band or working in a fashion department was her road to independence. It was a fantasy for which she worked very hard. By acquiring the clothes or accessories that helped create the desired image, she felt she was on her way to realizing her goal. In actuality, she had no work history at all. As noted above, work training for Sally placed her with other retarded persons which was a situation she could not tolerate.

Social Life: Sally's SDD worker described her as a loner, "sitting on the fence between the worlds of normalcy and the developmentally delayed." Sally felt she was persecuted and misunderstood. Even though she wanted good friends, she was difficult to get along with, extremely self-centered, and not well-liked by her peers at New Start. One of her roommates was Grace (of the Pseudo-Independents) who Sally referred to as a "dummy." Grace acknowledged that Sally did not like her but didn't care as she was still mad that Sally had forced her to sleep in the living room when they shared a New Start apartment.

Sally viewed retarded persons with profound disdain (her own IQ scores were in the high 60s). She preferred to associate with only the most normal-appearing New Start participants. On several occasions she shared her opinion that the people in New Start and at sheltered workshops were "retarded losers," to be avoided as much as possible.

During her two years in New Start she had three roommates, with whom she could not make friends. Her alienation from other New Start participants bordered on xenophobia.

When asked about other friendships outside the program she responded that there were ". . . not very many. Ever. I'd like more companions but somebody normal." Sally was caught between needing the approval of others and despising her natural peers.

Parental/Family Involvement: The SDD worker argued that the relationship between Sally and her mother contributed significantly to Sally's ambivalence about herself. Sally said:

> My mother tells me I am not retarded. I am emotionally handicapped and get frustrated easily when trying to find the right words to express my thoughts. I am very angry with my SDD worker because she told me I am retarded. I do not believe I am retarded.

The worker reported that Mrs. Redland had told Sally she could not afford to have her leave. "Mrs. Redland needs Sally's SSI income to help pay the rent because she is presently divorcing and without it, she would have to give up her apartment in a very desirable neighborhood. Her selfishness in demanding this from Sally obviously compounds Sally's conflicts about being independent."

Summary: The conspiracy of denial by Sally and her mother contributed much to Sally's development as the sheltered, unrisking, immature home-body. Their mutually reinforcing denial acted like an embalming fluid. Sally looked and acted like a permanently preserved teenage daughter. Beneath the carefully maintained image was an aging, frightened, retarded woman who was confused and demoralized. She owned a handicapped bus pass but re-fused to use it, electing to stay at home during the majority of her days where she was profoundly unhappy. The New Start program seemed incapable of addressing Sally's special issues and needs.

Pete Lippman

Appearance: Pete cultivated a young, sporty look; bright colors, clean white socks, name-brand tennis shoes, and clean, well-groomed hair. Physically, he was a visibly strong young man of average height, with a long face, curly hair, and bright, gleaming eyes. He looked quite normal.

Personal Background: Shortly after graduating from his special high school program, he made his first gesture to the world; he joined the Marines. Two months later he was released and back in his mother's home. By Pete's ac-count, he did not get along with the drill sergeant and he was unable to per-form certain tasks which required reading and math. He was proud that he got into the Marine Corps but also ashamed that he had failed to meet Corps expectations because he was born a slow learner.

Following the Marines setback, Pete enrolled in a bakery training program at his mother's suggestion. He had resisted the suggestion based on his sus-picion that the site where the training was to take place was for retarded and handicapped people. He assented once he learned that normal people also received vocational training there.

It was unclear whether he finished the bakery training program. How-ever, he acknowledged that he did not get along with his instructor, which at one point deteriorated into a shoving match.

Following the training, his mother made arrangements for Pete to work at a local bakery in Castleton, California, which was a small backroad town hundreds of miles away at the foot of the eastern Sierras.

Feeling that he was being exiled once again, he lost the bakery job within three weeks. He said he was too slow. However, he liked the town and was not ready to go home. He found work as a dishwasher, busboy and prep cook in a chicken restaurant and stayed eight more months.

Life in Castleton was not easy for Pete. He was a 21-year- old "flatlander," the slightly derogatory term locals reserve for the year-round parade of tourists and skiers. He did not have much of a social life and said he grew depressed. He had trouble paying his rent on time and returned to Los Angeles. Neverthe-less, he decided that, on the whole, his time in Castleton had been a success because he had been able to lose the job his mother set up for him, find another on his own, and rent his own apartment. By the time Pete returned from Castleton, both of his parents had remarried to spouses with normal children. The new children were living at home, so Pete had to be placed somewhere. Pete's mother found New Start.

From the beginning he fought going to New Start. By enrolling in the program he felt he was discrediting his successful Castleton experience. His parents applied great pressure to coerce his enrollment which he read as their lack of faith in him.

As a result, he entered New Start with a chip on his shoulder, determined to prove that New Start was beneath him. "When I first entered New Start I wished these places didn't even exist. Others don't fight like I do. They accept the special education. I refuse to accept it." In his mind, he had already proven he could make it on his own. He resolved to resist all attempts to demonstrate otherwise.

According to staff notes, when he entered the program, his functional skill levels were adequate. His two strengths were housekeeping and employability; his chief weakness was money management.

Pete was in Project New Start for only 18 months, four months less than the average. Only two other graduates in the sample finished in less time. Four things made Pete a notorious character at New Start: his continuous part-time employment which he secured on his own; his hobby of baking; his money management skills—poor budgeting with "creative" banking; and his sexual conquests.

Current Home Life: Two years after leaving New Start, Pete was 27 years old. In his own words, success meant having his own apartment, owning a car, making good money working at a job which interested him, and having a savings account of at least $1,000. These were not wishes; these were his minimum criteria for measuring his personal success. The only goal he had met was the $1,000 account.

Pete's return to his parents' homes was unplanned, apparently the direct result of his hastily arranged graduation from New Start. Pete's father asked the observer if Pete graduated from or was thrown out of New Start. Officially, he graduated, however, staff, parents, and Pete all agreed that the graduation came suddenly and unexpectedly. Pete said he was told to vacate his apartment so another resident could move in. No arrangements were made to place him in the community, which was unusual. He was allowed to discharge directly to his father's home.

He moved back into his mother's home about one year after leaving New Start. He had a part-time job at Goodwill "with the other losers," rode the bus or begged for rides, and was broke. He looked and sounded defeated.

By contrast, his home life in New Start had provided many daily pleasures attending to routine activities such as baking breads and muffins. He enjoyed mixing the batter, adding special ingredients not called for in the recipe (like raisins), kneading the dough, watching it rise, and, proudly removing his creation from the oven. He wanted to be a "sight baker" which he described as someone who could mix and bake without looking at a recipe or using measuring devices. Pete said:

> I use the recipe as a basic guide but also mainly put myself into it. I know how to do a lot of things by instinct, like how much water to add to rice, or what spice to add to this dish. I have picked up a lot of cooking skills and I don't always rely on recipes. I make mistakes, too. I am not perfect.

The concept of "sight-baking" appealed to Pete for two reasons: the idea of working free of reliance on tools or the advice of others; and his belief that to bake this way indicated mastery.

Money management was recognized by both Pete and New Start as his chief weakness. Prior to entering New Start he did not use a bank. Difficulties he had encountered paying rent on time were not due to lack of funds, however, but rather to poor budgeting. Pete tended to spend impulsively, especially on food.

At the market, he was a chronic budget-buster. He was observed during one of his first program-directed shopping trips. Although he spent twice his allotment, he was not outwardly concerned. He concluded that he had simply purchased food for two weeks instead of one. Nine months later he was still exceeding his food budget.

As impulsive as he was shopping for food, he was equally thrifty in other ways. Pete's money management system did not originate with the New Start program. It was his own plan that neatly sidestepped his weak check-balancing skills without costing him convenience, dollars, or security. He kept a savings account at the bank and cashed paychecks at the market. He explained that using the market instead of a bank made dollars and sense. At the market there were no account fees or minimum balance requirements and money orders cost 25 cents less than at his bank. Besides he preferred carrying cash ("about $40") and had eliminated his need for checks. Each month he wrote money orders for utilities and rent.

Personality: Pete usually made a strong first impression as he was not shy. Among the characteristics one immediately recognized were his confidence, his need to establish himself as knowledgeable, and his desire to be the leader. He made regular eye contact and would comment on many topics, eager to share an opinion. He also acknowledged when he was not well informed on a particular subject.

He could be quite funny with his self-righteous demeanor. For example, during a marketing observation he provided a running list of his do's and don'ts on food selection. He was a self-proclaimed "health food nut." He examined every item carefully. Produce had to show "a strong and natural color." Packaged foods had to be clean, containers undamaged in any way, and properly labeled for nutritional value. With all this in mind, he picked up a can of Dinty Moore Beef Stew in the middle of his monologue and fruitlessly searched its sides for the nutritional specifications. With true horror he proclaimed, "A can without a nutrition calendar on it...lacks dignity!"

Depressed was not a term that fit Pete's personality; robust was more like it. He loved challenges, and he hated being classified as handicapped, retarded, developmentally delayed, specially educated, or any other name which, in his words, simply meant outsider. "It is like they are telling me you go with this crowd. This is your speed."

Labeling angered him greatly, but also seemed to deepen his conviction and motivation to pursue his favorite goals and activities (for example, eating health food, weightlifting, or becoming a "sight-baker").

For Pete, success and revenge were interrelated. Being able to prove to others he could achieve his most ambitious or most modest goal was the sweetest revenge. Success vindicated him while simultaneously punishing his detractors.

Pete's immaturity was concealed by his great motivation and feelings of righteous anger. He was driven to prove that he was capable of living a full, normal life. He recognized that he was retarded, but was equally convinced that he was unlike other handicapped people; that he didn't belong with them. There was a direct relationship between the intensity of his anger and the lofty goals he often set for himself. His self-righteous pursuit of these goals led to folly on a grand scale.

Employment: One of his part-time jobs while in New Start was in a health food store which had a small food service area. As in Castleton, he washed dishes and cleared tables. He was eventually released from the job for unknown reasons. Back in his mother's home, he made about $300/month working part-time at Goodwill. He continued his pattern of getting into conflicts with supervisors. He had already found himself embroiled in a dispute with his Goodwill supervisor over the use of free passes to a show. He no longer received SSI.

Pete had lost and regained his SSI benefits at least twice. Each time he lost the benefit it was because he insisted on reporting his part-time employment earnings. He was the only subject interviewed in this sample who did not purposely attempt to conceal any extra income. For Pete, it was a matter of pride. Receiving SSI connoted failure to Pete and disproving that was more important to him than securing the benefits to which he was entitled.

Pete valued money greatly and was quite thrifty when he had to be. He could go into financial hibernation when needed, spending next to nothing for long periods of time. After graduating New Start he disclosed that he had $1,000 in a special savings account and $500 in his living expenses account. Seventeen months later he reported having $100 in his living expenses account and the same $1,000 in the other account.

Social Life: Since moving back to his parents' homes he had failed to make any friends or develop any social life. He said he was depressed. By contrast, he had been quite popular at New Start. It was rumored he had slept with several New Start women residents. With an air of chivalry, he would not elaborate on the rumors. At New Start, men and women who wished to live together were counseled to wait, but encouraged to go ahead with making plans to share a place after graduation. On the other hand, single men and women who simply wished to be sexually active were discouraged. Pete's casual sexual relations with participants were seen as a problem for staff.

Parental/Family Involvement: Pete was in public school when his parents divorced. Pete said that his father abandoned his mother and four children. His mother promptly removed Pete and his brother from her home. His brother was sent to live with an uncle in Wyoming and Pete was placed in a psychiatric residence with a special school. He had lived with his father on two occasions since. His father seemed disinterested in Pete's future.

Summary: One always had the distinct impression that Pete did not belong in New Start. Of course, Pete cultivated and nurtured this idea. Of greater significance was the evidence that Pete did not seem to belong anywhere. His father had left him behind twice, and his mother had sent him away twice.

Although he had shown determination in securing work at every turn, he had also lost every job he ever had, many times the result of conflict with an authority. He had failed to properly complete at least three training programs (baking, New Start and the USMC). By most appearances, his life was a complete failure.

On our last visit his spirit seemed crushed. "I never go out and have zero friends. For the past 12 months I have stayed home, watched TV, and slept. Then I did it all again the next day. That has been my whole day for a year. I quit lifting weights and eating health foods," Pete said

Ultimately, Pete believed he was to blame for his developmental delays. Such dark thoughts dominated his mood once he returned to his parents' homes. In contrast, his money management scheme was a prime example of his inventiveness and ability to adapt. Although Pete's program-identified weakness was his poor money management skills, in fact, he had rendered the problem insignificant in his own unorthodox way. Since leaving the New Start program, he had run out of either opportunities or interest to continue his struggle to live on his own terms.

Pete carried an enormous burden around with him. It included being stigmatized by the label of retardation, being rejected by his parents, and being cognizant of his own failure to complete a program. He had all the tools, apparently, to lead a normal, productive life. He was articulate, charming, sociable, courteous, strong-willed, ethical, and hard-working, to mention a few of his qualities. He was also stubborn, contrary, and somewhat conceited.

Ironically, his personal pride predisposed him to resist the support of others. He hated the implication that he needed help; that he was handicapped; that he was an outsider. He knew better than to let others know he was different in those ways. "I never mention that to them. I try to pass as though it's not even a question. I am afraid of what they might think if they knew. They might think I was dumb, a moron, a reject, stupid, from the scrap heap of life," Pete confided.

SECTION SUMMARY:
THE FAILURES

These three individuals who failed to establish any semblance of independent living were more similar than different in circumstances that appear to have contributed to their unhappy situations. Although one had a formidable work history, none were working by the time they left the New Start program. Pete had secured part-time work at Goodwill, but had already gotten himself into a dispute with his supervisor, a life-long pattern for Pete. Their contact with New Start after graduation was minimal, but not necessarily by design. Ernie had unsuccessfully tried to establish a regular contact, while Pete and Sally had tried to avoid contact with not only staffpeople but also other people with retardation.

Each of the three deplored being labeled retarded or handicapped. Their reactions to labeling ranged from comparatively mild (in the case of Ernie), to indignant (Pete), to outright denial (Sally and her mother). None had significant incomes. Ernie was dependent on his mother's trust account which his father administered. Sally received SSI which her mother appropriated as her rent contribution. Any assessment of Pete's relationship with SSI had to take into account his pride, his history of being disqualified so many times, and his belief that he didn't deserve it because he was capable of working. In short, none of the subjects could rely on a fixed income which they controlled even though each demonstrated as much capability as any other subject in handlng money.

Sally claimed to be the most socially active, although indicators showed she imagined a more active, exciting, and satisfying social calendar than actually existed. Pete and Ernie, like Sally, were equally charming but without longstanding friendships. Neither of them made any friends in the program which continued beyond graduation. In the cases of all three, friendship was something they all cherished and desired. The absence of friends surely contributed to their feelings of depression, which all three shared.

Finally, the role of their parents was confusing. The parents of both Pete and Ernie seemed to provide support grudgingly. Pete's parents preferred to place him outside their homes, if at all possible. When forced to harbor him in their homes, they bounced him back and forth between them like an unwanted visitor. The effect on Pete's self-esteem was devastating.

Ernie could not possibly replace his protective, psychologically enmeshed mother. His father retained control of Ernie's trust but also made it clear to Ernie that after his move to Arizona he would be unavailable. It is fair to conclude that, given the condition of Ernie's home, his father must never have visited or, if he did, felt unmoved to provide simple guidance in terms of hygiene and housekeeping. Ernie felt alone in the world.

Sally's mother, who was also an enmeshed parent, divorced the father while simultaneously drawing Sally closer. She supported the conspiracy of denial and told Sally she needed her SSI check to survive. Sally was given minimal chores around the house and was prohibited from contributing to the home or family in other ways. She was her mother's prisoner.

This group held some of the brightest promise among all the subjects. Pete and Ernie shared the intelligence, enthusiasm, and many of the resources which helped Walter and Stefan succeed. Sally should have been at least as successful as Darlene. Their failures in the face of their special talents was especially disappointing.

In the least, their failures illustrated that success could not be described in a simple formula: neither a function of IQ, previous institutionalization, mental illness, size of the program, the program philosophy itself, nor two year's worth of assessment and instruction in banking, cooking, and house-cleaning.

Chapter 7

Implications for Training in Independent Living

Conclusions from this study are presented in three sections. First, standards for assessing successful independent living, based upon the descriptions of graduates, are discussed. Second, programmatic issues which may have had an impact on the success of graduates, and very likely contributed to the program's deterioration, are presented. Third, concluding remarks and recommendations are explored.

STANDARDS OF SUCCESS FOR INDEPENDENT LIVING

There is an implicit association between prediction and quantitative approaches to understanding community adaptation. Academic literature on the subject is steeped in this tradition. It has been argued here, and by others, that quantified approaches have yielded little understanding.

It is now argued that prediction, as a quantitative method, also comprises an inadequate approach to the phenomenon as it presumes that success and failure are fixed and static outcomes. Results of this research have shown that success and failure in community adaptation of people with mild mental retardation must be understood phenomenologically; as a changing, variant, idiosyncratic event, a function of the individual in the context of personal history and learning environment.

Instead of isolating variables which may or may not predict a person's ability to live independently, the description of interpersonal relationships, external circumstances, life experiences, and the individual's own understanding of successful independent living may lead to greater understanding of success and failure. As these phenomena change so might an individual's status as a success or failure at living independently.

Findings for this study were phenomenological, rather than quantitative. For example, placing the subjects into separate but similar subgroups was a preliminary finding. Three categories of success—the Independents, the Pseudo-Independents, and the Failures—were proposed based upon the observations of each sample member, and discussed under seven subheadings: appearance, personal background, current home life, personality, employment, social life, and parental/family involvement.

With respect to appearance, the Independents were each noticably different physically even though they blended well with the normal population. Their personal backgrounds varied widely. The issue of labeling was not a damaging stigma for any of them. Their current home lives were marked by privacy and independence with respect to the management of their own funds and their separation from formal support agencies, especially New Start. Walter and Stefan enjoyed strong social lives which were not dependent on either their families or associations for the retarded.

The personalities of all three varied a great deal, however, none evidenced significant, debilitating psychopathology. Each individual was highly motivated to become independent. Janice, Randy, Stefan and Walter had strong work histories and high skill levels vis a vis the traditional areas of independent living skills instruction. Finally, all except Janice held the reins of control with regard to their parents' roles in their lives. Janice shared that control with her mother, and only she appeared to have a somewhat enmeshed relationship with a parent.

The Pseudo-Independents also tended to have physical features that drew attention to them, however, their benign demeanors generally helped them to pass unnoticed by others. Their personal backgrounds varied as to the circumstances which brought them to New Start. A great number, though not all, felt coerced by circumstances and/or relatives to enroll. For example, Ernie lost his mother suddenly. He focused his resistance to enrolling in New Start on securing a guarantee from his father that he would be able to return to his home once he graduated. Grace and Ida also lost parents (who lived full lives) which forced the inevitable arrangements for their continued care to be made. Darlene's mother remarried and informed her she would no longer be able to care for her daughter in the home.

Francis Larsen's alcoholism and subsequent unmanagable behavior contributed to his removal from his board and care home, forcing placement in an alternative site, New Start. June LePoap's sister persuaded June to enroll as she could not continue to watch over her because of marital difficulties. On the other hand, Aileen and Kristy seemed to have been placed in New Start as part of their parents' plan to train their daughters to live on their own.

Their current home lives featured privacy in living arrangements and secure incomes, but only Darlene controlled the management of funds. For all but the Larsens and Darlene, this arrangement was preferable. Their living skills levels varied, but as a rule were adequate. The level of psychopathology was noticably greater within this group. Four of the subjects (Francis, June, Aileen and Ida) had significant personality problems including alcoholism, physically abusive relationships, and extreme psychological dependency which were regularly indulged in dealings with others. However, like the Independents, they accepted their mental retardation label without apparent conflict.

They did not possess the ambition of the Independents and in fact as a group seemed content with their present status in life. They had poor work histories which many did not wish to improve. They tended to be much more involved with their parents, other family members, and agency or agency-related staff than the Independents.

Their parents controlled the family relationships, which were clearly enmeshed in the cases of Aileen and June. Ida, who had a highly enmeshed relationship with both her parents, bred enmeshed relationships with everyone she encountered, including Grace. Even Darlene, who had the most distance in her relationship with her mother, suffered from a moderately enmeshed relationship with a parent. The relationship between the Larsens and Francis' cousin Roy also featured the resentment and dependency of enmeshed psychology. Finally, most of the members in this subgroup had active daily schedules and some sort of social life.

The Failures were the most normal-looking subjects in the sample; they dressed and behaved in such a way that they quietly passed for normal (even Ernie when he was relatively clean). They were also among the youngest subjects. Two of the three were clearly coerced into entering New Start. All three had lost, or were about to lose, contact with a parent which may have contributed to their lack of direction in life. All three lived at home, although Ernie had inherited the home. Two of them were quite bitter and angry about being labeled.

This bitterness was prominent in their personalities and their personal lives. None enjoyed successful social lives although each wanted one very badly. All three were clinically depressed. Only Pete had a good work history, although his personality repeatedly figured in his dismissal from jobs. Each was quite immature in their psychological development. Ernie's and Pete's parents were reluctantly involved in their son's life.

Sally's mother was deeply enmeshed with her daughter. In Sally's case, her mother's denial of Sally's retardation was especially damaging to Sally's development. Unlike the Independents or the Pseudo-Independents, the Failures received marginal financial assistance from their parents, even though two of them lived with their parents.

The sole trait which all three groups shared was their inability, or their reluctance, to either balance or learn to balance their own checkbooks.

The effect that being part of a couple has on success, and the nature of psychopathology and an enmeshed familial relationship as it relates to success, bears further discussion. Eight of the subjects were paired as couples; two married, and two platonic relationships. All four couples met and made their bonds after they entered the New Start program. The two platonic couples were roommates in the program. Not everyone may benefit from a couple relationship, however, in the cases of these eight participants the pairings seemed to have significantly improved their chances for success.

For example, Ida and Grace were able to at least temporarily ameliorate their psychosocial deficits (Ida's irritating dependency, and Grace's cool silence) by providing constant companionship for each other. Walter and Stefan were able to practice and polish their skills in social leadership, building confidence and sharing the limelight. Later, both young men utilized these skills on their own to develop independent social lives.

The Larsens developed limited but effective escapes from their controlling family relationships. Finally, the Daltons matched strengths with weaknesses: his ability to work and earn a regular income with her contagious enthusiasm.

The practice of fostering couples merits consideration as a possibly significant addition to programming in community residential facilities. In the cases of these four couples, the pairings were either initiated on their own, as with the married Larsens and Daltons, or were effected almost at random in that no formal policy which placed a premium on fostering couples existed within the program. Ida had already had two roommates before she was placed with Grace. The matching of Walter and Stefan, according to the two men, was effectively by chance.

While all New Start residents were paired with someone, the criteria for making the matches had as much to do with staff and program convenience as with any other factor. Placing the emphasis on personality traits which portend compatibility and opportunity for personal growth in a fostered partnership certainly deserves consideration equal to program convenience.

Along with the successful pairings there were numerous examples of failed matches. In particular, Ernie and Pete were especially ill-matched. In both cases, they were matched with another young man who added little if anything to each other's personal development. In Ernie's case, being placed with a diagnosed schizophrenic left him without a role model which, because of his immaturity, he desperately needed. Pete, who possessed a strong personality, saw himself as highly ethical, and valued health foods and good physical condition, was placed with a physically disabled young man who regularly smoked marijuana and seemed mostly concerned with circumventing the program's rules. Both Ernie and Pete gained little if anything from their New Start experiences.

It seemed clear that the fostering of friendships (which sometimes develop into romance) was a worthwhile endeavor for program staff and program participants. Friendships should have been fostered with care; nurtured thoughtfully. Participants were often ill-matched. This effect could have been monitored closely and intervention made immediately.

The meaning of psychological disturbance in people with mental retardation has been an issue of some controversy. Kernan, et al. (1978), stated that the isolation of mental health issues as predictors of failure was a sign of bias against people with retardation. The history of researchers' efforts to characterize them as psychologically dangerous or unpredictable was too much like a self-fulfilling prophecy. Kernan and his colleagues cited numerous studies which found that the retarded were markedly impaired by a significantly higher incidence of personality disorder. As discussed in Chapter 2, the earliest literature on people with mental retardation was rife with references to this theme.

Despite the discouraging signs, researchers have continued to explore the relationship of psychosocial characteristics and psychiatric or emotional disturbance in regard to this population. Levine's (1985), and Levine and Langness's (1985) work on performance anxiety described the psychological underdevelopment of people with mild mental retardation from a primarily social perspective.

Linden and Forness (1986) addressed the psychological side of this issue by describing the additional difficulty which "dual-diagnosed" (having both a mental retardation and a psychiatric diagnosis) retarded people have in adjusting to the community. Matson (1984) has advocated that psychotherapy should be an integral component in any program that seeks to enable community adjustment for people with mental retardation.

Zetlin and Turner (1985) argued the point that individuals with retardation can be raised within a family system that may not contribute to successful personal growth and may, in fact, obstruct such development. As they put it, the awareness of limitations by the person (as reinforced in the family through excessive caretaking) "may lead to feelings of dissonance and be expressed in behavioral and emotional problems."

Complex psychosocial phenomena, such as personality disorder or psychological dysfunction, was noted within this sample. Records of 14 of the 15 subjects showed evidence of suicidal ideation, psychotropic medication, or psychiatric histories. Nevertheless, five of the subjects were considered to be clearly successful and seven others nearly successful. The simple presence or absence of psychopathological manifestations did not appear to be a determinant of successful independent living in this sample.

However, the presence of enmeshed family relationships clearly seemed to be instrumental in the developmental delays of many subjects. The interaction of psychopathology and relationships with others, such as key family members or members of program staff, merits further understanding within the context of each individual's success.

Zetlin and Turner's categories described general adjustment patterns during the adulthood years of their sample. Zetlin and Turner's more psychological view was tested with these subjects by seeing how well the categories fit this sample. Independent adults (almost half their sample) were those who "handled most of the everyday affairs of their lives without assistance" or support from their parents except "in times of crisis." All were proud of their "independence and self-sufficiency. . . less involved in and dependent on delivery system support and agency counselors."

Almost all were employed, either competitively or in sheltered situations, and had large friendship circles. The five sample members from this study (one third of the total sample) who fell into the mostly successful group, also called the Independents, met many of Zetlin and Turner's criteria. All but one worked; had generally supportive but non-interfering relationships with their parents; counted on and received financial support from their parents in crisis situations which for this group ran the gamut from loss of work by layoff, to loss of income from an SSI dispute, to the loss of a roommate by murder.

One key difference was that, within this sample, only two roommates, Walter and Stefan, enjoyed wide-ranging and satisfying friendship circles. The other couple felt isolated and lonely, while the single woman, Janice, whose roommate was murdered, claimed no friends at all. In fact, her life was marked by transience in work, friendships, and living space until her parents bought her a condominium in a very exclusive, low-crime area. Janice was fierce in her independence, and enjoyed her parent's considerable support financially and emotionally, both of which seemed to help compensate for her somewhat unstable behavior that was reflected in her poor interpersonal skills and job transience.

Zetlin and Turner's Dependent adults "looked to their parents for protection and guidance in virtually every dimension of their lives. Both parents and the retarded adults viewed this as necessary and desirable. . .These members were also heavily enmeshed in the service delivery system. . .were more socially immature. . .(some) were involved in unstable marriages."

The majority of this sample's members (seven) fell into this category as described by Zetlin and Turner. As Dependents, these seven subjects lived independently in name with the help of a constellation of key support persons. These often included family members whose involvement may have contributed to their lower level of functional independence. In some cases such as Aileen and June, these parent/child relationships may have been fairly described as dysfunctional at some point in the past.

Only one member of this group, Francis Dalton, worked competitively; for his brother's fast food restaurant. All were financially dependent on their family or SSI. Most of them allowed a family member to manage or supervise their finances. None enjoyed friendships of any significance outside the key family member. Most of their social interactions centered around their daily routines of appointments or tasks to be accomplished with the help of, or in response to a request by, support persons. In each case, the involved family member was viewed as essential to their continued independence.

In addition to the family member, there were almost always agency counselors or medical doctors extensively involved. These members regarded and identified themselves as independent, but were in fact dependent on many. More significantly and perhaps more likely, was that this group did not know how to make friends.

The three sample members from this study who comprised the Failures possessed qualities much like Zetlin and Turner's Interdependent adults who were "enmeshed in conflict-ridden relationships with parents," soliciting assistance from their parents while resenting their dependence on that support.

In turn, the parents "preferred less involvement but insisted on maintaining control over decisions affecting their child's life." These individuals were unemployed, although one had a checkered employment history marked by conflict with supervisors. Each had an enmeshed parent; for two the parent was reluctant to offer assistance, regarding their adult child as an unfortunate nuisance. For the other, the relationship with her parent was purely dysfunctional with a complete denial of handicap and constant acting-out behavior on the part of both the parent and the adult child. As Zetlin and Turner found, these persons were regarded by service workers as "manipulative and unchangeable."

It is clear that the role of the family deserves thorough and continual attention in the evaluation of a candidate for independent living training. Furthermore, investigation of the extent to which dysfunctional relationships contribute to the failure of apparently good candidates seems worthwhile. Finally, one must wonder how much the mere introduction of a child with retardation into a family has to do with the likelihood that dysfunction, or more specifically, an enmeshed parent/child involvement will develop within the family.

PROGRAMMATIC ISSUES THAT IMPACTED PARTICIPANTS' SUCCESS

The programmatic issues which follow relate to the four internal conditions discussed in Chapter 3: staff turnover; program evaluation policy; staff supervision practices; and the role and effect of a prominent leader.

Staff Turnover

New Start administrators attempted to cast the chronic problem of frequent staff turnover in a positive light. Since staff turnover was unavoidable (as confided by a former director of HOK) New Start chose to view itself as a stepping-stone for young professionals entering the field of human services. Most employees were expected to leave New Start within a couple of years, either to return to school or to accept a position of greater responsibility, or greater pay, within the same field.

When Mr. Mickelson left New Start to become the director of SDD he became the best example of fulfilling the New Start employment dream: to move up in responsibility and income within the same field. However, employment history data for all HOK staff suggest that Mickelson's case was the exception rather than typical, and that the actual incidence of staff career moves, either laterally or upward, was low.

In addition, there was a generally worsening problem at HOK: an accelerating turnover rate. Staff were not only leaving the agency in greater numbers, but also after shorter durations of employment. As reported by Halpern et al. (1984), annual turnover rate can be a measure of program stability. The calculation as commonly practiced loses meaning, however, when the number of available staff positions changes drastically during a given year, as was the case in virtually every year for the growing New Start program. Nevertheless, the idea of a ratio which reflects program stability is useful, and the turnover rate can be adapted to the New Start situation in order to illustrate an important point.

Staff turnover has been a chronic problem with CRF's. From a survey of forty-four CRF's in four Western states, Halpern (1985) indicated that annual staff turnover rates of more than 50 percent were common. Turnover rate should be considered within the context of staff qualifications (i.e., the standards for hiring staff), another area which varied widely at New Start. Despite an impressive number of staffpeople with degrees (nearly 80 percent of the program counselors held at least a bachelor's, which was considerably higher than the rate observed by Halpern, 1985), one director commented that "our staff is limited by age, experience, and pay; no question." Many staff fit the image of the young helping professional working at the agency to gain valuable experience.

However, there were other employees who were clearly not committed to the field and offered little to the program. One director complained that he was limited by budgetary constraints. He could offer counselors only a $12,000 annual salary. Office space was minimal. He felt it was a given that every employee would eventually leave New Start, usually sooner than later. He described employees as being one of three types: 1.) people in flux with school or jobs; 2.) good people from bad agencies; and 3.) people who have stagnated in their careers and bounce from one job to the next.

The combination of a high rate of staff turnover and poor incentive to stay on the job eventually worked to discourage the well-qualified employees from remaining on staff. Staff burnout became a problem of major significance without remedy. Despite the presence of qualified staffpeople, the supervision and instruction of program participants was inconsistent, at least in part, due to the instability of the staff. While it cannot be demonstrated that this inconsistency impeded success, it is suspected that it did not enable it. A New Start senior counselor described how this phenomenon affected his job:

> Here is the problem. There is too much staff turnover to ever get a consistent program going. The constant changes in staff and, lately administrators, cuts off any momentum that can be generated. On the other hand, change may be endemic to this operation. We may never be stable. In the last year we have had three directors. In the first year I was here there was only one but she burned out and fell apart. On the other hand there were still alot of counselors coming and going.

Program Evaluation Policy

The widespread practice among service programs to use detailed assessment instruments has been criticized by Bercovici (1984). She points out two inherent problems: 1.) the possible failure of form-based ratings to reveal causes for apparent individual or program deficiencies; and 2.) the tendency for low scores in specific areas to become prescriptions for treatment.

Informants for this study suggested that the use of the Blue Form and the Followup Form (survey instruments adapted internally from a generic model) was the primary and, effectively, the sole form of evaluation practiced at New Start. One counselor stated "our evaluation instruments are really inappropriate for the people. Many of the items are inapplicable, especially the hygiene and grooming ones, and on the whole, the tools are too broad; (they are) geared to lower functioning MRs." A second counselor commented that he used the evaluation tool in lieu of staff training. By reading it carefully he felt better informed on the particulars of task-analysis for the basic skills of money management, cooking, shopping, and housekeeping.

Bercovici (1984) suggested that effective evaluation for this population has previously failed to consider the context in which behavior was found. "While it is undoubtedly important to recognize the areas in which the individual will have difficulties with certain norms of the mainstream culture, it is not sufficient to see these as merely deficiencies. A more complete evaluation should include a consideration of the situation to which a particular behavior pattern may be an adaptive response (p.166)."

Assigning the task of evaluation to someone untrained in methodology was a poor administrative decision. The absence of an adequate evaluation program or policy prohibited cohesive formulation and subsequent assessment of program goals and objectives. It also compromised the identification of carefully considered criteria for measuring the participant's successful program completion within a relevant context. Instead, New Start relied on the completion of two forms, both of questionable reliability and validity, to evaluate program effects.

Staff Supervision

As a program, New Start was dependent on its counselors to deliver at a minimum adequate services to the participants. Comments by persons interviewed for this study suggested that staff may have been unclear as to their proper role with the participants. One of the agency's directors believed that the counselors were "afraid of how to develop a relationship with the client, as educator or counselor."

One senior counselor described the method of becoming a New Start counselor as seat-of-the-pants. "We are 50 percent teachers and 50 percent therapists. I have become a lay therapist by doing this work. But we have no training in that." All these phenomena have been described by Fimian (1984) as typical of community-based programs characterized by disorganization and poor delivery of services.

Weekly group and/or individual sessions between counselors and senior or consulting staff to discuss issues of programmatic and personal concern (such as identification of training needs, or delineation of clear role boundaries) comprise one typical supervisory format. Inservice sessions are another form of supervisory practice commonly found in human service agencies. Both forms of supervision occurred at New Start, although their incidence was described either as infrequent, irregular, or inadequate.

The low incidence of formal training and supervision appeared to necessitate the staff's dependence on their own instincts, personal backgrounds, and nascent beliefs about what they considered to be programmatically correct. Trina, for example, was a counselor recruited from the agency's clerical staff. The site director felt she possessed qualities which made her especially empathic in her brief but daily encounters with the clients as office secretary. She was a 31-year-old, single woman who wished to advance professionally. She was promoted to counselor on the condition that she would pursue her bachelor's degree.

As a counselor, she quickly became known as "Drill Sergeant," a nickname she earned for her rigid adherence to program rules, such as making a client remove steak and shrimp from his shopping list because they were not on his weekly meal plan.

During a separate interview, the director spoke about how there was a problem of staff antagonizing parents. "I sometimes suspect that there is more at play than meets the eye. It often feels that there is a very personal struggle going on between some of our young counselors and the families of their clients, as though our counselors are working on their own family struggles with these clients' families."

The controversial incident in which Trina was involved with Aileen's parents (referred to earlier in Chapter 3) was a case in point. She felt she had to prove that Aileen had lied and stolen. The Karnan's did not believe Trina's contention that Aileen had been using old food receipts to conceal pinching money from her grocery budget in order to increase her dining out budget.

Trina's personal anger with the parents was obvious. She faulted them for making Aileen look retarded in the clothing they chose for her. She also was angry that, although the Karnans were professional educators, their daughter was so manipulative and immature. The episode raised the issue of staff prejudice in working with their clients. Such issues would have fallen squarely within the domain of those to be addressed during individual or group staff supervisory training sessions.

The problem of staff involvement with clients and families is normal for any direct-service program. A typical strategy for teaching young counselors to remain effective and avoid counterproductive behavior (referred to clinically as countertransference) is to have the counselors work regularly on their feelings with a skilled leader in a training group. Such a format would have provided Trina with the chance to recover from her apparent overreaction, instead of developing more entrenched biases. Unfortunately, staff supervision took place irregularly at best for New Start staff. According to the senior counselor the need was great, and unmet:

> We meet with the staff psychologist twice a month. This is not enough. We need more and it needs to be a different format. We usually end up talking about one or two cases and not about our own personal issues with the clients. And for a pretty counselor like Trina the issues of sexual attraction are always present but seldom explored among staff. The sexual innuendos or contacts between clients and counselors, a touch here and a word there, are really sticky and need to be discussed. These are examples of the kinds of things that are never discussed, or seldom discussed, and that make a big difference in a counselor's work. The whole question of proper role is important and not clearly defined for the counselors. The problem of being too buddy-buddy or too aloof is a continuous one.

Without formal and regular supervision, staff were left to draw their own conclusions about what did and did not work with their clients. A set of beliefs and principles emerged for the counselors in the absence of supervised experience. For example, Trina viewed the client/counselor relationship as adversarial. She believed that clients would go to great lengths to avoid doing what they should. She said that she had learned to distrust the clients. As an example, she related that program participants would say they understood an instruction, such as how to complete a bank transaction, yet they would make the same mistake over and over.

The senior counselor spoke of the same phenomenon, although in more forgiving and educational terms. Nevertheless, he was also speaking about not being able to take the clients at their word. For him it was "too easy to assume that the clients could understand the simplest discussion. Even the simplest discussion could not be assumed to be understood."

Formalized staff supervision, such as that found in clinical mental health settings, would have provided an opportunity to anticipate the difficulties typically encountered by novice counselors; e.g., learning to contend with their own psychological dynamics as well as those of their clients.

The senior counselor captured his own frustration concerning his lack of preparedness.

> We need training. We are just thrown into this job. It is assumed that because we brush our teeth with no thought that it might be an easy task to teach. Well, it isn't. Too often the client has a difficult time understanding the task and we simply rescue them for expedience's sake...First of all we need a better understanding of the population we are working with. I don't think we really understand them as a group. We cannot assume they will learn with the same ease we do.

The Role and Effect of a Prominent Leader

Mr. Mickelson was the first and longest-standing executive for HOK and Project New Start. As such, his character had a tremendous impact on the agency's performance, just as his personal style shaped his own career development.

Three informants provided an insider's view on the man and his style. It must be pointed out that discussion of the New Start executive as an example of how a leader affected a small social service agency was largely conjectural and not conclusive. However, the data obtained provided the opportunity to make some interesting speculations about his impact on the program.

Mickelson helped New Start prosper in many ways. He greatly increased the client and staff rosters. He had a far-reaching effect on both the staff (promoting the agency as a place to develop careers), and the clients. His contributions to the program were easily documented. On the other hand, there was evidence that could not be ignored which suggested that his management style and his personal ambition may have affected New Start detrimentally.

For example, Mickelson doubled his salary to well over $30,000 during his tenure. Halpern's data showed that executive directors at 44 Western region SILP's (including New Start) earned salaries averaging in the mid $20,000s. It was not clear whether Mickelson's exceptional salary was more a reflection of his performance at New Start or of his considerable influence with the HOK governing board who would have to approve salary increases for the executive.

His personal charisma was exceptional and may have been a factor in the changing turnover rate by keeping turnover low when the agency was small and his personal contact with staff was more frequent. When the agency grew and his personal focus shifted to personal career advancement, his charismatic influence over the staff may have diminished. The degree to which Mickelson delegated hiring authority to his immediate subordinates, especially during the key years when staff size doubled and redoubled, may have also contributed to staff turnover, subsequently impacting the program negatively.

His career interests appeared to have eventually conflicted with his administrative functions. In the program's earlier years his personality may have been more useful to operations as his charisma and ambition helped increase program enrollment. In the latter years, when the program needed leadership to manage its unregulated growth and overburdened staff, the same factors may have proved to be handicaps. The program's rapid downfall, which coincided with his sudden departure from New Start and arrival as director of the SDD, suggested that his personality, rather than effective management skills, carried the program for many years.

CONCLUDING REMARKS AND
RECOMMENDATIONS

At Project New Start, skill building was considered by most staff and support agencies to be essential in teaching clients how to become independent. The learning of skills, however, did not correspond to successful independent living. There was no apparent relationship between the broad teaching of traditional living skills and demonstrated independent living success in this study.

Banking was a skill few subjects mastered, while doing laundry was a skill everyone could perform. Self-management of funds (with or without checkbook balancing), however, was a trait which distinguished the Independents from the rest. Cooking, housekeeping, etc., varied widely within each criterion group, apparently unrelated to successful lifestyle. In fact, most subjects exited the program at the same skill levels as when they entered. The assumption that the teaching and learning of these skills was a precursor to successful independence and therefore should have been the foundation of training programs, should be questioned.

As previously discussed, the success of the couples within this sample was viewed as a significant finding. The practice and art of matchmaking represented an important area of investigation for training programs and a reasonable goal in program planning. The process of identifying these participants and making the best match should be a part of staff development in current programs.

Program participants were not the only consumers of program services. In this study, one could often view the entire family system as a program participant. As such, the needs and dynamics of the entire family system should be addressed in the design of an effective living skills program.

If the purpose of programs like New Start is to provide the most normalizing experience to its participants in order to elicit and maintain normalized behaviors, then the parents must be included in the normalization process. Parents or siblings who were enmeshed with the participants often became obstacles to normalization. On the other hand, certain parents managed to keep a distance yet still provide critical financial and emotional support. Often in these cases, the distance had to do with a willingness to stand aside for the most part from their adult child's decisions to take on risk in life. The careful assessment of these relationships (friends, parents, siblings, service agency staff) by the program staff may be the single most important factor in designing successful training for independent living.

The manner in which a program is conceptualized and subsequently administered has a direct bearing on the likely success of its participants. In this study, participants who graduated during New Start's early years, (i.e., by mid-1982) fared better. These would include Walter and Stefan, and Janice. The three graduates included among the Failures all began in mid-1982 and graduated in 1984 (Pete in late 1983). The long-time director left the agency amid wide disarray in late 1983.

In retrospect, many of the subjects seemed to possess ample abilities and talents to make life on their own an attainable goal. In the cases of many of the Independents and Pseudo-Independents, specific aspects of their personalities or their family relationships were overlooked or misperceived and, as a result, not integrated into their program plans. Nevertheless, all of these subjects were able to establish independent living situations. For the Failures, the inability of either the program or the basic approach to training people with mental retardation to address these needs, resulted in these particularly capable and resourceful individuals being simply thought of as unsuccessful graduates.

Special attention must be paid to the group of seven subjects called the Pseudo-Independents. Their lives are precariously perched on the two pillars of fixed income and a carefully self-constructed, often enmeshed, network of service workers and family. They seem especially vulnerable, therefore, to national economic hardship, professional matriculation, and the good will of personal relationships. Their self-styled success is a plateau from which they seek no further advancement. This presents policymakers, service providers, and researchers with a new group to consider as part of the changing population of people with mild retardation adapting to independent life in the community.

References

Aininger, M., and Bolinsky, K. (1977). Levels of independent functioning of retarded adults in apartments. *Mental Retardation, 15,* 12-13.

Alkin, M.C. (1978). A new role for evaluators. *CSE Monograph Series in Evaluation (No. 97).* Los Angeles: Center for the Study of Evaluation, University of California.

Alkin, M.C. (1981). *Evaluation use in local schools.* Paper presented at the Fiftieth Annual Conference of the American Educational Research Association, Los Angeles, April.

Alkin, M.C., Daillak, R., and White, P. (1979). *Using evaluation: Does evaluation make a difference?* Beverly Hills, CA: Sage Publications.

Anderson, V.V. (1922). Feeblemindedness as seen in court. *Boston Medical and Surgical Journal, 176,* 429-431.

Baker, B.L., Seltzer, G.B., and Seltzer, M.M. (1974). *As close as possible.* Boston: Little Brown & Co.

Baldwin, N.F. (1978). *Adaptive behavior changes of mentally retarded citizens in community residences.* Paper presented at the Annual Meeting of the American Psychological Association, Toronto, Canada.

Balla, D.A. (1976). Relationship of institution size to the quality of care: A review of the literature. *American Journal of Mental Deficiency, 81,* 117-124.

Beier, D.C. (1964). Behavioral disturbances in the mentally retarded. In H.A. Stevens and R. Heber (Eds.), *Mental Retardation: A Review of Research.* Chicago: University of Chicago Press.

Bercovici, S.M. (1978). *The deinstitutionalization of mentally retarded persons: ethnographic research in community environments, Working Paper No. 3.* Los Angeles: Socio-Behavioral Group, University of California.

Bercovici, S.M. (1981). Qualitative methods and cultural perspectives in the study of deinstitutionalization. In R.H. Bruininks, C.E. Meyers, B.B. Sigford, and K.C. Lakin (Eds.), *Deinstitutionalization and Community Adjustment of Mentally Retarded People, AAMD Monograph No. 4* (pp.133-144). Washington, D.C.: American Association on Mental Deficiency.

Bercovici, S.M. (1983). *Barriers to normalization.* Baltimore: University Park Press.

Bishop, E.B. (1957). Family care: The patients. *American Journal of Mental Deficiency, 61,* 583-591.

Bjaanes, A.T., and Butler, E.W. (1974). Environmental variation in community care facilities for mentally retarded persons. *American Journal of Mental Deficiency, 78,* 429-439.

Bogdan, R., and Taylor, S.J. (1976). *Introduction to qualitative research methods: A phenomenological approach to the social sciences.* New York: John Wiley & Sons.

Boruchow, A.W., Espenshade, M.E. (1976). A socialization program for mentally retarded young adults. *Mental Retardation, 14,* 40-42.

Brown, D.L. (1952). The working convalescent care program for female patients at Rome State School. *American Journal of Mental Deficiency, 56,* 643-654.

Brown, S.J., Windle, C., and Stewart, E. (1959). Statistics on a family care program. *American Journal of Mental Deficiency, 64,* 535-542.

Bruininks, R.J., Kudla, M.J., Hauber, F.A., Bradley, K., and Wieck, C.A. (1981). Recent growth and status of community residential alternatives. In R.H. Bruininks, C.E. Meyers, B.B. Sigford and K.C. Lakin (Eds.), *Deinstitutionalization and Community Adjustment of Mentally Retarded People, AAMD Monograph No. 4* (pp. 14-27). Washington, D.C.: American Association on Mental Deficiency.

Bruininks, R.J., Kudla, M.J., Wieck, C.A., and Hauber, F.A. (1980). Management problems in community residential facilities. *Mental Retardation, 84,* 470-478.

Butler, E.W., and Bjaanes, A.T. (1977). A typology of community care facilities and differential normalization outcomes. In P. Mittler and J. deJong (Eds.), *Research to Practice in Mental Retardation: Care and Intervention, (Vol. 1).* Baltimore: University Park Press.

Butterfield, E. (1976). Some basic changes in residential facilities. In R.B. Kugel and A. Shearer (Eds.), *Changing Patterns in Residential Services for the Mentally Retarded.* President's Commission on Mental Retardation. Washington, D.C.: U.S. Government Printing Office.

Cobb, O.H. (1923). Parole of mental defectives. *Proceedings of the American Association for the Study of the Feebleminded, 28,* 145-148.

Crnic, K.A., and Pym, H.A. (1979). Training mentally retarded adults in independent living skills. *Mental Retardation, 17,* 13-16.

Cronbach, L.J. (1975). Beyond the two disciplines of scientific psychology. *American Psychologist, 30.*

Dingman, H.F. (1967). *A plea for social research in mental retardation. American Journal of Mental Deficiency, 73,* 2-4.

Duker, P.C., van Druenen, C., Jol, K., Oud, H. (1986). Determinants of maladaptive behavior of institutionalized mentally retarded individuals, *American Journal of Mental Deficiency, 91,* 51-56.

Eagle, E. (1967). Prognosis and outcome of community placement of institutionalized retardates. *American Journal of Mental Deficiency, 72,* 232-243.

Edgerton, R.B. (1967). *The cloak of competence: stigma in the lives of the mentally retarded.* Berkeley: University of California Press.

Edgerton, R.B. (1977). The study of community adaptation: Toward an understanding of lives in process. In P. Mittler and J. deJong (Eds.), *Research to Practice in Mental Retardation: Care and Intervention, (Vol. 1).* Baltimore: University Park Press.

Edgerton, R.B. (1988). Aging in the community: A matter of choice. *American Journal on Mental Retardation, 92,* 331-335.

Edgerton, R.B. and Bercovici, S.M. (1976). The cloak of competence: Years later. *American Journal of Mental Deficiency, 80,* 485-497.

Eisner, E. (1981). On the differences between scientific and artistic approaches to qualitative research. *Educational Researcher, 10* (4), 5-9.

Eyman, R.K., Demaine, G.C., Lei, T. (1979). Relationship between community environments and resident changes in adaptive behavior: A path model. *American Journal of Mental Deficiency, 83,* 330-338.

Feldman, A. (1946). Psychoneurosis in the mentally retarded. *American Journal of Mental Deficiency, 51,* 247-254.

Fernald, W.E. (1919). After-care study of the patients discharged from Waverly for a period of twenty-five years. *Ungraded, 5,* 25-31.

Fernald, W.E. (1924). Thirty years progress in the care of the feebleminded. *Journal of Psycho-Asthenics, 29,* 206-219.

Fimian, M.J. (1983). Organizational variables related to stress and burnout in community-based programs. *Education and Training of the Mentally Retarded, 19,* (3), 201-209.

Fimian, M.J., Santoro, T.M. (1983). Sources and manifestations of occupational stress as reported by full-time special education teachers. *Exceptional Children, 49,* 540-543.

Fondacaro, M.R., Heller, K., Reilly, M.J. (1984). Development of friendship networks as a prevention strategy in a university megadorm. *The Personnel and Guidance Journal, 62* (9), 520-523.

Freedman, R. *A study of the community adjustment of deinstitutionalized mentally retarded persons. Vol. 1.* Approaches to defining and measuring the community adjustment of mentally retarded persons: A review of the literature. Cambridge, MA: Abt Associates (Contract No. OEC-0-74-9183, U.S. Office of Education).

Fritz, M., Wolfensberger, W., and Knowlton, M. (1971). *An apartment living plan to promote integration and normalization of mentally retarded adults.* Downsview, Ontario: Canadian Association for the Mentally Retarded.

Gage, N. L. (1989). The paradigm wars and their aftermath: A "historical" sketch of research on teaching since 1989. *Educational Researcher, 18* (7), 4-10.

Garrison, K.C. and Force, D.G., Jr. (1965). *The Psychology of Exceptional Children (4th ed.).* New York: Ronald Press.

Goddard, H.H. (1909). Suggestions for a prognostic classification of mental defectives. *Journal of Psycho-Asthenics, 14,* 48-54.

Gollay, E. (1976). *A study of the community adjustment of deinstitutionalized mentally retarded persons. Vol. 1.* Approaches to defining and measuring the community adjustment of mentally retarded persons: A review of the literature. Cambridge, MA: Abt Associates (Contract No. OEC-74-9183, U.S. Office of Education).

Guba, E.G. (1978). Toward a methodology of naturalistic inquiry in educational evaluation. *CSE Monograph Series #8,* UCLA.

Halpern, A.S., Close, D.W., and Nelson, D.J. (1986). *On my own: The impact of semi-independent living programs for adults with mental retardation.* Baltimore: University Park Press.

Hanrahan, J., and Lusthaus, E. (1978). *Preparing mildly retarded young adults for integration into the community: Observations on quality of life.* Paper presented at the World Congress on Future Special Education.

Heal, L.W., Sigelman, C.K., and Switzky, H.N. (1978). Research on community residential alternatives for the mentally retarded. In N.R. Ellis (Ed.), *Research in Mental Retardation, Volume 9* (pp.210-249). New York: Academic Press.

Heller, K., Rasmussen, B.R., Cook, J.R., Wolosin, R. (1981). The effects of personal and social ties on satisfaction and perceived strain in changing neighborhoods. *Journal of Community Psychology, 9* (1), 35-44.

Hill, B.K., Lakin, K.C. (1986). Classification of residential facilities for individuals with mental retardation. *Mental Retardation, 24,* 107-115.

Hirsch, E.A. (1959). The adaptive significance of commonly described behavior of the mentally retarded. *American Journal of Mental Deficiency, 63,* 639-646.

Hull, J.T., and Thompson, J.C. (1980). Predicting adaptive functioning of mentally retarded persons in community settings. *American Journal of Mental Deficiency, 85,* 253-261.

Hutchisson, D.A. and Rush, V.M. (1983). *The process of adjustment of developmentally disabled adults and their families to an independent living situation.* Unpublished master's thesis.

Hutt, M.L., and Gibby, R.G. (1965). *The Mentally Retarded Child (2nd. ed.).* Boston: Allyn and Bacon.

Johnson, B.S. (1946). A study of cases discharged from Laconia State School from July 1, 1924 to July 1, 1934. *American Journal of Mental Deficiency, 50,* 437-445.

Johnson, G.O. (1963). Psychological characteristics of the mentally retarded. In W.M. Cruikshank (Ed.), *Psychology of Exceptional Children and Youth (2nd. ed.).* Englewood Cliffs, NJ: Prentice Hall.

Kernan, K.T., Turner, J.T., Langness, L.L., and Edgerton, R.B. (1978). *Issues in the community adaptation of mildly retarded adults, working paper no. 4,* Los Angeles: Socio-Behavioral Group, University of California.

King, T., Soucar, E., and Isett, R. (1980). An attempt to assess and predict adaptive behavior of institutionalized mentally retarded clients. *American Journal of Mental Deficiency, 84,* 406-410.

Lakin, K.C., Bruininks, R.H., and Sigford, B.B. (1981). Perspectives on the community adjustment of mentally retarded people. In R.H. Bruininks, C.E. Meyers, B.B. Sigford, and K.C. Lakin (Eds.), *Deinstitutionalization and Community Adjustment of Mentally Retarded People, AAMD Monograph No. 4* (pp.28-50). Washington, D.C.: American Association on Mental Deficiency.

Landesman-Dwyer, S., Berkson, G., Romer, D. (1979). Affiliation and friendship of mentally retarded residents in group homes. *American Journal of Mental Deficiency, 83,* 571-580.

Langone, J., Burton, T.A. (1987). Teaching adaptive behavior skills to moderately and severely handicapped individuals: Best practices for facilitating independent living. *The Journal of Special Education, 21* (1) 149-165.

Levine, H.G. (1978). *Everyday problem-solving in a school for children with moderate retardation.* Paper presented at the 77th Annual Meeting of American Anthropological Association in Los Angeles, California.

Levine, H.G. (1985). Situational anxiety and everyday life experiences of mentally retarded adults. *American Journal of Mental Deficiency, 90,* 27-33.

Levine, H.G. and Langness, L.L. (1985). Everyday cognition among mildly mentally retarded adults: An ethnographic approach. *American Journal of Mental Deficiency, 90,* 18-26.

Lewin, K. (1936). *A dynamic theory of personality,* New York: McGraw-Hill.

Linden, B.E. and Forness, S.R. (1986). Post-school adjustment of mentally retarded persons with psychiatric disorders: A ten-year follow-up. *Education and Training of the Mentally Retarded, 21* (3), 157-164.

Macmillan, M.B. (1962). Adjustment and process: A neglected feature of follow-up studies of retarded people. *American Journal of Mental Deficiency, 67,* 418-430.

Madison, H.L. (1964). Work placement success for the mentally retarded. *American Journal of Mental Deficiency, 69,* 50-53.

Matson, J.L. (1984). Psychotherapy with persons who are mentally retarded. *Mental Retardation, 22* (4), 170-175.

McCarver, R.B. and Craig, E.M. (1973). Placement of the retarded in the community: Prognosis and outcome. In N.R. Ellis (Ed.), *Research in Mental Retardation, Volume 7.* New York: Academic Press.

McKay, B.E. (1942). A study of IQ changes in a group of girls paroled from a state school for mental defectives. *American Journal of Mental Deficiency, 46,* 496-500.

McPherson, G.E. (1935). Parole of mental defectives. *Proceedings of the American Association on Mental Deficiency, 40,* 162-176.

Morrissey, J.R. (1966). Status of family-care programs. *Mental Retardation, 4* (5), 8-11.

Mundy, L. (1957). Environmental influence on intellectual function as measured by intelligence tests. *British Journal of Medical Psychology, 30,* 194-201.

Nirje, B. (1976). The normalization principle. In R.B. Kugel and A. Shearer (eds.), *Changing Patterns in Residential Services for the Mentally Retarded.* President's Commission on Mental Retardation. Washington, D.C.: U.S. Government Printing Office.

O'Connor, N. (1957). The successful employment of the mentally handicapped. In L.T. Hilliard and B.H. Kirman, (Eds.), *Mental Deficiency* (pp.448-480). London: Churchill, Ltd.

Patton, M.Q. (1978). *Utilization focused evaluation.* Beverly Hills: Sage Publications.

Pratt, M.W., Luszcz, M.A., and Brown, M.E. (1980). Measuring dimensions of the quality of care in small community residences. *American Journal of Mental Deficiency, 85,* 188-194.

Procidano, M.E., Heller, K. (1983). Measures of perceived social support from friends and from family: three validation studies. *American Journal of Community Psychology, 11* (1), 1-24.

Rhoades, C.M., Browning, P.L., Thorin, E.J. (1986). Self-help advocacy movement: a promising peer-support system for people with mental disabilities. *Rehabilitation Literature, 47* (1-2), 2-7.

Roos, P., Patterson, E.G., and McCann, B.M. (undated, ca. 1970). *The developmental model.* Arlington, Texas: National Association for Retarded Citizens.

Rossi, P.H., Freeman, H.E., and Wright, S.R. (1979). *Evaluation: A systematic approach.* Beverly Hills: Sage Publications.

Rossi, P.H., and Wright, S.R. (1977). Evaluation research: An assessment of theory, practice, and politics. *Evaluation Quarterly, 1.*

Sarason, S.B., and Gladwin, T. (1958). Psychological and cultural problems in mental subnormality. In R.L. Masland, S.B. Sarason, and T. Gladwin (eds.), *Mental Subnormality.* New York: Basic Books.

Scriven, M. (1973). Goal-free evaluation. In E. House (Ed.), *School Evaluation: The Politics and Process.* Berkeley: McCutcheon.

Seltzer, M.M. (1985). Informal supports for aging mentally retarded persons. *American Journal of Mental Deficiency, 90,* 259-265.

Shafter, A.J. (1954). The vocational placement of institutionalized mental defectives in the United States. *American Journal of Mental Deficiency, 59,* 297-307.

Shafter, A.J. (1957). Criteria for selecting institutionalized mental defectives for vocational placement. *American Journal of Mental Deficiency, 61,* 599-616.

Skeels, H.M., and Dye, H.A. (1939). A study of the effects of differential stimulation on mentally retarded children. Proceedings of the *American Association on Mental Deficiency. 44,* 114-136.

Slater, M.A., Bunyard, P.D. (1983). Survey of residential staff roles, responsibilities, and perception of resident needs. *Mental Retardation, 21,* 52-58.

Smith, J.K. (1983). Quantitative versus qualitative research: An attempt to clarify the issue. *Educational Researcher, 12* (3), 6-13.

Stake, R.E. (1972). The case study method in social inquiry. Educational Researcher, 7 (2), 5-8.

Stainback, W., Stainback, S. (1987) Facilitating friendships. *Education and Training in Mental Retardation, 22* (1), 18-25.

Sternlicht, M. (1978). Variables affecting foster care placement of institutionalized retarded residents. *Mental Retardation, 16,* 25-28.

Sullivan, C.A.C., Vitello, S.J., and Fosters, W. *ETMR, 23* (1), 76-81.

Sutter, P., Mayeda, T., Call, T., Yanagi, G., and Yee, S. (1980). Comparison of successful and unsuccessful community-placed mentally retarded persons. *American Journal of Mental Deficiency, 85,* 262-267.

Tarjan, G., Dingman, H., Eyman, R., and Brown, S. (1959). Effectiveness of hospital release programs. *American Journal of Mental Deficiency, 64,* 609-617.

Taylor, S.J. and Bogdan, R. (1977). A phenomenological approach to mental retardation. In B. Blatt, D. Biklen, and R. Bogdan (Eds.), *An Alternative Textbook in Special Education* (pp.193-204). Denver: Love Publishing Co.

Taylor, J.R. (1976). A comparison of the adaptive behavior of retarded individuals successfully and unsuccessfully placed in group living homes. *Education and Training of the Mentally Retarded* (pp.56-74).

Tizard, J. (1960). Residential care of mentally handicapped children. *British Medical Journal, 1,* 1041-1046.

Tymitz, B. and Wolf, R. (1977). *An introduction to judicial evaluation and natural inquiry.* Nero and Associates (Mimeo).

Wallace, G.L. (1929). Are the feebleminded criminals? *Mental Hygiene, 13,* 93-98.

Wallin, J.E.W. (1924). *The education of Handicapped Children (Part 3).* Boston: Houghton.

Weiss, C.H. (1970). The politicization of evaluation research. *Journal of Social Issues, 26* (4), 57-68.

Weiss, C.H. (1972). Utilization of evaluation: Toward comparitive study. In C.H. Weiss (Ed.), *Evaluating Action Programs: Readings in Social Action and Education* (pp.318-326). Boston: Allyn and Bacon.

Windle, C.D. (1962). Prognosis of mental subnormals. *American Journal of Mental Deficiency, 66,* (Monograph Supplement).

Windle, C.D., Stewart, E., and Brown, S. (1961). Reasons for community failure of released patients. *American Journal of Mental Deficiency, 66,* 213-216.

Wolfensberger, W. (1977). The principle of normalization. In B. Blatt, D. Biklen, and R. Bogdan (Eds.), *An Alternative Textbook in Special Education* (pp.305-328). Denver: Love Publishing Co.

Wolfensberger, W. (1972). *The Principle of Normalization in Human Services.* Toronto: National Institute on Mental Retardation.

Wyngaarden, M., and Gollay, E. (1976). *A study of the community adjustment of deinstitutionalized mentally retarded persons. Vol. 2.* Profile of national deinstitutionalization patterns 1972-1974. Cambridge, MA: Abt Associates (Contract No. OEC-0-74-9183, U.S. Office of Education).

Zetlin, A.G., and Turner, J.L. (1985). Transition from adolescence to adulthood: perspectives of mentally retarded individuals and their families. *American Journal of Mental Deficiency, 89,* 570-579.

Zigler, E. (1976). *Effects of preinstitutional history and institutionalization on the behavior of the retarded.* Lectures presented for Meyer Children's Rehabilitation Institute, University of Nebraska Medical Center, Omaha, NE.

About the Author

Steven H. Stumpf, Ed.D. trained in Research Methods and Evaluation at the UCLA Graduate School of Education. This manuscript was developed from his doctoral dissertation.

Dr. Stumpf works in two professions: program evaluation and clinical psychotherapy. Currently he works as a program evaluator for the Physician Assistant program at the University of Southern California School of Medicine. He also maintains a private practice in psychotherapy in West Los Angeles.

"Endlessly fascinated and moved" by the human spirit, he finds that improving the quality of life often follows a pattern of identification, recognition, anticipation and intervention. It is the application of this model that challenges most persons and organizations every day.